Clinician's Manual on Migraine

Todd A. Smitherman

Clinician's Manual on Migraine

Adis

Todd A. Smitherman
Department of Psychology
The University of Mississippi
Oxford, MS
USA

ISBN 978-3-319-02776-0 ISBN 978-3-319-02777-7 (eBook)
DOI 10.1007/978-3-319-02777-7

Library of Congress Control Number: 2016938002

Printed on acid-free paper

This Adis imprint is published by Springer Nature
The registered company is Springer International Publishing AG Switzerland

To my sister, Laura

Preface

This handbook details the assessment and evidence-based treatment of migraine in adults. Migraine is the third most common medical condition worldwide but is often underdiagnosed and insufficiently treated in clinical settings. This handbook incorporates diagnostic criteria from the most recent edition of the International Classification of Headache Disorders, third edition (ICHD-3), as well as recently published reviews on evidence-based pharmacotherapy. It is not intended to be a comprehensive overview of the entire field of headache medicine or all possible methods of care, but rather a concise clinical guide. This guide is intended for healthcare professionals who work with migraine and other headache patients, including primary care physicians, neurologists, emergency room physicians, and behavioral health providers.

The information herein is based on assessment of current scientific literature, including published treatment guidelines, meta-analyses, and randomized controlled trials. Because several of the pharmacologic agents with empirical support are used off-label for migraine, some off-label drug use is reviewed insofar as it is supported by empirical evidence or clinical guidelines. Individual patient care decisions must ultimately occur between the patient and the treating provider.

Note: Because migraine occurs disproportionately in women, the feminine pronoun "she" is used throughout this book.

Oxford, MS, USA Todd A. Smitherman

Contents

Author Biography

Todd A. Smitherman, PhD, FAHS is an Associate Professor of Psychology and Director of the Center for Behavioral Medicine at the University of Mississippi. He has published over 65 peer-reviewed journal articles, numerous book chapters, and one other book, most of which focus on primary headache disorders and behavioral factors associated with these conditions. His research has been supported by grants from the Migraine Research Foundation, the American Headache Society, the University of Mississippi, and Merck Pharmaceuticals. Dr. Smitherman serves as Associate Editor for the journal *Headache: The Journal of Head and Face Pain*, is a Fellow of the American Headache Society and past Chair of its Behavioral Issues Section, and serves on the Common Data Elements Working Group for Headache Clinical Trials for the National Institute of Neurological Disorders and Stroke.

Chapter 1
Introduction

1.1 Definition

Migraine is a common medical condition characterized by recurrent episodes of moderate to severe head pain lasting hours or days and accompanied by other associated symptoms [1]. The head pain is usually throbbing or pulsatile in nature and experienced unilaterally (on one side of the head) and commonly accompanied by nausea, vomiting, or sensitivity to both light (photophobia) and sound (phonophobia). The presence of the latter symptoms conveys that migraine is far more than a typical "headache." Because of the high pain severity and other debilitating symptoms, migraine attacks frequently interfere with activities of daily living, and patients experiencing migraine (migraineurs) often seek respite in a low-stimulus environment such as a dark quiet room.

A significant minority of migraineurs will experience aura symptoms, which are sensory abnormalities that precede the onset of head pain and then resolve. Most often, the aura symptoms are visual in nature (e.g., seeing spots or lights, fortification spectra, zigzag lines) that gradually expand unilaterally across the visual field; occasionally aura symptoms may present as temporary alterations in speech or motor functioning.

Episodic migraine (EM) refers to migraine attacks that occur fewer than 15 days per month (with or without aura).

T.A. Smitherman, *Clinician's Manual on Migraine*,
DOI 10.1007/978-3-319-02777-7_1,

This subsumes the large majority of individuals with migraine, as most will have attacks 1–4 days per month [2]. A very small proportion of patients with migraine experience chronic migraine (CM), in which headache attacks occur at least 15 days per month on average for at least 3 months, most of which have features of migraine. CM thus denotes migraine characterized by abnormally high attack frequency.

1.2 Prevalence and Impact

Data from the World Health Organization indicate that migraine is the third most prevalent medical condition in the world, affecting 14.7 % of the population annually [3]. In the largest US-based, migraine-specific population study to date, the American Migraine Prevalence and Prevention (AMPP) Study observed an annual prevalence of 11.7 % when using strict adherence to International Classification of Headache Disorders (ICHD) diagnostic criteria [2]. Somewhat higher rates have been observed in other national government surveillance studies that have used different criteria [4, 5]. Overall, it has been found that migraine affects women three times more often than men (17.1 % vs. 5.6 %), whites more than blacks, and those of low income more than those of higher socioeconomic status [2]. Prevalence is high during young and middle adulthood, peaking between ages 30 and 39, during which time 28.1 % of women and 9.0 % of men will experience migraine. Prevalence declines precipitously after middle age and is lowest among adults 60 and older. In the United States, the prevalence of CM is approximately 1 %, and these individuals make up a large portion of treatment-seeking headache patients [6].

The overwhelming majority of migraineurs (92.5 %) experience at least some impairment during migraine attacks, and for 53.7 % of patients, severe functional impairment occurs (i.e., bed rest is required). Because of this high prevalence and burden, migraine is ranked as the eighth leading cause of disability worldwide (i.e., years lived with disability), placing it ahead of diabetes, osteoarthritis, and alcohol and drug abuse disorders [3]. Migraine represents the fourth leading cause of visits to the emergency department, where one out of every six outpatient visits for migraine occurs [4].

1.3 Risk Factors and Triggers

Risk factors for developing migraine de novo include the presence of common comorbid conditions, a family history of migraine, and being female, given that migraine has a significant genetic component and that women experience migraine more than men [2]. In large part, this gender discrepancy stems from hormonal influences, as migraine is commonly triggered by dramatic fluctuations in estrogen levels, such as those that occur during menstruation, the first trimester of pregnancy, and perimenopause. Many women will experience migraine only around the time of menstruation ("menstrual migraine"), while others will have migraine attacks around menstruation and also during other times of the year ("menstrually related migraine"). Risk of migraine is increased ±2 days before or after menstruation.

Migraine "triggers" are personal or environmental events that precipitate individual headache attacks among those who have migraine. Most migraineurs endorse having multiple triggers, as most triggers do not occasion a migraine upon every exposure. The most commonly reported triggers of migraine are stress, hormonal changes (in women), skipping or missing meals (fasting), and inadequate sleep, all of which are reported by at least 50 % of migraineurs [7]. Other common triggers include weather changes, strong smells, visual factors (e.g., lights, glare), drinking alcohol (particularly red wine), cigarette smoking, and exercise. Many patients also report that particular food items are triggers, most commonly aged cheeses, monosodium glutamate (MSG), caffeine, and chocolate. However, studies have not always confirmed the potency of these dietary triggers, and the mechanisms responsible for food-induced headaches are both variable and incompletely understood.

Triggers may also interact with one another. For example, an individual who is under significant stress often obtains inadequate sleep, portending a greater risk for migraine than exposure to either trigger alone [8]. Much of the uncertainty surrounding the causal nature of headache triggers stems from a preponderance of retrospective versus experimental studies, as well as difficulty simultaneously controlling for numerous variables that can influence the individual and triggers over time [9].

1.4 Comorbidities

Although migraine per se is not associated with increased risk for all-cause mortality, migraine is associated with increased risk for other medical conditions, in particular cardiovascular disease, seizures, sleep disruption, and mood disorders [10, 11]. These comorbid conditions account for a large portion of role disability experienced by migraineurs and may complicate diagnosis and treatment [12].

Data from meta-analyses indicate that migraine is associated with a doubled risk for ischemic stroke but only among those who have migraine with aura [13, 14]. The risk is highest for women who use oral contraceptives and smokers. A risk for subclinical white matter lesions also has been linked to migraine [15]. A relationship between obesity and CM is well established [16].

Migraine and epilepsy both are chronic neurological conditions with episodic attack manifestations, and the risk for having one and later developing the other is approximately doubled among individuals who have one of these conditions [17]. The migraine–epilepsy relationship is bidirectional in nature, suggesting shared underlying mechanisms [17].

Insomnia is the most common sleep disorder among individuals with migraine and presents as recurrent difficulty initiating or maintaining sleep with accompanying daytime impairment (e.g., restlessness, anxiety, trouble concentrating, fatigue). Insomnia often goes unrecognized in migraineurs but affects over half of those who seek treatment for migraine and over 80 % of those with CM. Sleep apnea is also common among migraineurs, particularly those who are overweight or obese. Waking in the morning with headache is often suggestive of a contributing sleep disorder, and treating the underlying sleep disorder often reduces migraine frequency.

Psychiatric disorders commonly co-occur among individuals with migraine, particularly major depressive disorder and anxiety disorders such as panic disorder, post-traumatic stress disorder, and phobias [18, 19]. Compared to those without migraine, migraineurs are between two and four times more likely to be diagnosed with these psychiatric disorders. Increased rates of bipolar disorder and personality disorders have also been observed [18, 20], particularly among those presenting to specialty clinics. Conflicting evidence exists regarding whether migraineurs are at increased risk for substance use disorders. Prevalence of psychiatric disorders is highest among migraineurs with aura, patients with CM, and those who seek treatment in specialty clinics or are refractory to standard treatments [21]. As with epilepsy, these relationships appear bidirectional in nature, potentially suggestive of shared etiology, such as serotonergic dysfunction. Importantly, these psychiatric comorbidities are risk factors for overuse of acute headache medications and increasing headache frequency over time.

1.5 Prognosis

Migraine per se is not fatal, and most EM sufferers can self-manage their condition by making needed lifestyle changes such as maintaining a consistent sleep schedule, eating regular meals, stress management, and occasional use of over-the-counter acute medications. Some patients will only require infrequent physician consultation and can often manage their attacks using a pharmacologic agent. Many migraineurs will experience a reduction of attacks over time, and some will have the condition resolve without any intervention. Those with more frequent attacks or attacks conferring substantial disability typically require more substantial intervention, including preventive pharmacologic and/or behavioral interventions in conjunction with judicious use of an acute migraine medication. Approximately 25 % of migraineurs merit daily preventive pharmacotherapy, but only half of these currently receive it [2], as migraine remains underdiagnosed and undertreated in clinical settings.

A small proportion of individuals with EM each year will experience a progressive increase in headache frequency and cross the threshold of 15 headache days per month to be considered CM. This phenomenon of increasing headache frequency from EM to CM is termed "headache chronification" and is estimated to occur among 2–3 % of migraineurs each year [22, 23]. (A much larger proportion of those with CM remit to EM annually, and the reported rates of both chronification and remission may be in part influenced by random measurement error [24].) Those with CM may improve with treatment and their headache frequency may fluctuate over time, but they are unlikely to become headache-free. Established risk factors for headache chronification include high baseline attack frequency, overuse of acute migraine medications, obesity, sleep-related breathing disorders, and psychological variables such as depression and stressful life events [25].

1.6 Pathogenesis

Although the pathophysiology of migraine is complex and incompletely understood, at its core migraine is thought to be attributable to a hypersensitive central nervous system (CNS) that has difficulty properly modulating normal sensory stimuli [26]. Traditionally, the vascular theory of migraine held that constriction and subsequent dilation of blood vessels in the head caused migraine, but that theory has since been discredited. Vascular changes do occur, but they are relatively unrelated to symptoms and treatment response and thus secondary to events at the CNS level.

Vulnerability to migraine is in part genetic, although the precise genetic influences of the most common forms of migraine are as yet unknown. According to the prevailing neurovascular model, migraine involves an interaction between the brainstem, the cortex, and the trigeminovascular system [26]. Dysfunction of brainstem regions involved in pain, such as the periaqueductal gray, impairs descending modulation of pain. Impairment in pain modulation is accompanied by cortical spreading depression (CSD), a wave of neuronal inhibition that travels from the occipital lobe to the front of the cortex and is the established cause of visual aura. (Whether CSD occurs in individuals without aura is not firmly established but has been suggested.) This wave of inhibition sensitizes the trigeminovascular system, and head pain is perceived once the meningeal afferents of the ophthalmic division of the trigeminal nerve are activated. This activation culminates in release of neuropeptides, dilation of innervated meningeal blood vessels, and neurogenic inflammation. Over time, repeated attacks further sensitize the brainstem, the cortex, and peripheral nociceptors, resulting in "central sensitization" that increases vulnerability for additional attacks, as well as related states of hypersensitivity, such as allodynia and hyperalgesia. Most recently, efforts have been made to incorporate limbic system influences into an understanding of migraine pathophysiology to better account for the emotional and psychological influences on migraine [27].

1.7 Stages of a Migraine Attack

While virtually all patients with migraine recognize the pain and other symptoms required for diagnosis, a significant proportion of migraineurs also experience other stages of migraine that precede or follow the acute episode. The stages of migraine are commonly termed premonitory, aura, headache, and resolution.

Premonitory (or prodromal) symptoms are those that typically precede the headache attack by several hours (or even up to 1 or 2 days). Accurate estimates of the prevalence of premonitory symptoms are unavailable, owing in large part to a lack of many prospective studies [28], but it is likely that a significant minority of migraineurs experience them. Common premonitory symptoms include anxiety, fatigue, repetitive yawning, neck stiffness, mood changes, gastrointestinal upset or appetite changes (loss of appetite, food cravings), and sensitivity to light and sound (without pain). Because symptoms are often subtle and may go unrecognized by the patient, it is important that clinicians inquire about premonitory symptoms. Becoming proficient at noting premonitory symptoms that are predictive of forthcoming migraine, such as through keeping a headache diary, provides opportunities to abort the attack.

Aura symptoms occur regularly among 25–30 % of migraineurs, and on occasion some patients will experience aura without subsequent headache. Most patients who have migraine with aura will also have some attacks without aura symptoms. Aura most commonly presents as a transient visual disturbance, such as fortification spectra, scintillating scotoma, or seeing spots or arcs of light, that develops gradually and lasts up to an hour, after which pain and other features of the headache episode commence. Occasionally patients have sensory aura symptoms (e.g., paresthesia, numbness), and even less frequently aphasic aura, but visual aura usually precedes these symptoms or occurs during their other migraine attacks.

The headache episode itself has been described previously, in which pain and accompanied features of nausea/vomiting, photophobia, and phonophobia are present for 4–72 h. (In children and adolescents, the duration may only be 2 or 3 h, and the pain is often bilateral.) Prototypically, the pain is experienced unilaterally and has a pulsing/throbbing quality, although attacks may include bilateral pain or a pressing/ tightening sensation. During severe episodes, bed rest is often required, as the patient may be unable to perform routine movements (e.g., bending over, climbing stairs) and normal levels of light and sound can aggravate the pain. Rarely, a debilitating migraine episode may continue unabated for more than 72 h ("status migrainosus"), and emergency medical care is indicated.

Some patients experience alterations in physiology and behavior after the headache episode has resolved. This stage of resolution or "postdrome" commonly involves symptoms from the premonitory phase as well as lethargy, feeling lightheaded or dizzy, or difficulty concentrating. Most commonly, this period of low energy and other symptoms resolves over several hours, though for some patients it may continue for 1 or 2 days.

References

1. Headache Classification Committee of the International Headache Society. The international classification of headache disorders. 3rd ed. (beta version). Cephalalgia. 2013;33:629–808.
2. Lipton RB, Bigal ME, Diamond M, Freitag F, Reed ML, Stewart WF; for the American Migraine Prevalence and Prevention Advisory Group. Migraine prevalence, disease burden, and the need for preventive therapy. Neurology. 2007;68:343–9.
3. Vos T, Flaxman AD, Naghavi M, et al. Years lived with disability (YLDs) for 1160 sequelae of 289 diseases and injuries 1990–2010: a systematic analysis for the Global Burden of Disease Study 2010. Lancet. 2012;280:2163–96.
4. Burch RC, Loder S, Loder E, Smitherman TA. The prevalence and burden of migraine and severe headache in the United States: updated statistics from government health surveillance studies. Headache. 2015;55:21–34.
5. Smitherman TA, Burch R, Sheikh H, Loder E. The prevalence, impact and treatment of migraine and severe headaches in the United States: a review of statistics from national surveillance studies. Headache. 2013;53:427–36.
6. Buse DC, Manack AN, Fanning KM, et al. Chronic migraine prevalence, disability, and sociodemographic factors: results from the American Migraine Prevalence and Prevention Study. Headache. 2012;52:1456–70.

7. Kelman R. The triggers or precipitants of the acute migraine attack. Cephalalgia. 2007;27:394–402.
8. Houle TT, Butschek RA, Turner DP, Smitherman TA, Rains JC, Penzien DB. Stress and sleep duration predict headache severity in chronic headache sufferers. Pain. 2012;153:2432–40.
9. Turner DP, Smitherman TA, Martin VT, Penzien DB, Houle TT. Causality and headache triggers. Headache. 2013;53:628–35.
10. Åsberg AN, Stovner LJ, Zwart JA, Winsvold BS, Heuch I, Hagen K. Migraine as a predictor of mortality: the HUNT study. Cephalalgia. 2015. [Epub ahead of print].
11. Schürks M, Rist PM, Shapiro RE, Kurth T. Migraine and mortality: a systematic review and meta-analysis. Cephalalgia. 2011;31:1301–14.
12. Saunders K, Merikangas K, Low NCP, Von Korff M, Kessler RC. Impact of comorbidity on headache-related disability. Neurology. 2008;70:534–47.
13. Mawet J, Kurth T, Ayata C. Migraine and stroke: in search of shared mechanisms. Cephalalgia. 2015;35:165–81.
14. Schürks M, Rist PM, Bigal ME, Buring JE, Lipton RB, Kurth T. Migraine and cardiovascular disease: systematic review and meta-analysis. BMJ. 2009;339:b3914.
15. Kruit MC, van Buchem MA, Hofman PAM, et al. Migraine as a risk factor for subclinical brain lesions. JAMA. 2004;291:427–34.
16. Chai NC, Scher AI, Moghekar A, Bond DS, Peterline BL. Obesity and headache: part I – a systematic review of the epidemiology of obesity and headache. Headache. 2014;54:219–34.
17. Haut SR, Bigal ME, Lipton RB. Chronic disorders with episodic manifestations: focus on epilepsy and migraine. Lancet Neurol. 2006;5:148–57.
18. Baskin SM, Smitherman TA. Migraine and psychiatric disorders: comorbidities, mechanisms, and clinical applications. Neurol Sci. 2009;30 Suppl 1:S61–5.
19. Breslau N. Psychiatric comorbidity in migraine. Cephalalgia. 1998;18 Suppl 22:56–61.
20. Davis RE, Smitherman TA, Baskin SM. Personality traits, personality disorders, and migraine: a review. Neurol Sci. 2013;34 Suppl 1:7–10.
21. Buse DC, Silberstein SD, Manack AN, Papapetropoulos S, Lipton RB. Psychiatric comorbidities of episodic and chronic migraine. J Neurol. 2013;260:1960–9.
22. Bigal ME, Serrano D, Buse D, Scher A, Stewart WF, Lipton RB. Acute migraine medications and evolution from episodic to

chronic migraine: a longitudinal population-based study. Headache. 2008;48:1157–68.
23. Scher AI, Stewart WF, Ricci JA, Lipton RB. Factors associated with the onset and remission of chronic daily headache in a population-based study. Pain. 2003;106:81–9.
24. Houle TT, Turner DP, Smitherman TA, Penzien DB, Lipton RB. Influence of random measurement error on estimated rates of headache chronification and remission. Headache. 2013;53:920–9.
25. Bigal ME, Lipton RB. Modifiable risk factors for migraine progression. Headache. 2006;46:1334–43.
26. Goadbsy PJ, Charbit AR, Andreou AP, Akerman S, Holland PR. Neurobiology of migraine. Neuroscience. 2009;161:327–41.
27. Maizels M, Aurora S, Heinricher M. Beyond neurovascular: migraine as a dysfunctional neurolimbic pain network. Headache. 2012;10:1553–65.
28. Maniyar FH, Sprenger T, Monteith T, Schankin CJ, Goadsby PJ. The premonitory phase of migraine: what can we learn from it? Headache. 2015;55:609–20.

Chapter 2
Diagnosis and Clinical Evaluation

2.1 Migraine Diagnostic Criteria

All headache disorders, including migraine, are diagnosed according to the criteria specified in the International Classification of Headache Disorders, which is currently in its third edition (ICHD-3), and the tenth edition of the World Health Organization's International Classification of Diseases (ICD-10) [1, 2]. ICHD-3 diagnostic criteria for episodic migraine with and without aura are shown in Table 2.1.

Migraine without aura is the most common headache diagnosis among treatment-seeking individuals with headache as their chief complaint. Prototypically, migraine presents as severe head pain that lasts several hours, interferes with usual activities, or prompts bed rest and is accompanied by nausea or made worse by normal levels of both light (photophobia) and sound (phonophobia). Vomiting occurs among only 30 % of migraineurs. In younger adults and in patients with very frequent headache attacks, such as those with chronic migraine (CM), prototypical migraine features are less common [3].

Aural symptoms occur in 25–30 % of migraineurs and usually present as transient visual distortions that develop gradually over 5–20 min, last less than an hour, and then are followed by onset of head pain. When transient motor

T.A. Smitherman, *Clinician's Manual on Migraine*, DOI 10.1007/978-3-319-02777-7_2,

TABLE 2.1 Diagnostic criteria for episodic migraine

Migraine without aura (ICHD-3 1.1)	
A. At least five attacks fulfilling criteria B–D	
B. Headache attacks lasting 4–2 h (untreated or unsuccessfully treated)	
C. Headache has at least of the two following characteristics:	Unilateral location Pulsating quality Moderate or severe pain intensity Aggravation by or causing avoidance of routine physical activity (e.g., walking or climbing stairs)
D. During headache at least one of the following:	Nausea and/or vomiting Photophobia and phonophobia
E. Not better accounted for by another ICHD-3 diagnosis	
Migraine with aura (ICHD-3 1.2)	
A. At least two attacks fulfilling criteria B and C	
B. One or more of the following fully reversible aura symptoms:	Visual Sensory Speech and/or language Motor Brainstem Retinal
C. At least 2 of the following characteristics:	At least one aura symptom spreads gradually over ≥5 min, and/or two or more symptoms occur in succession Each individual aura symptom lasts 5–60 min At least one aura symptom is unilateral[a]
D. Not better accounted for by another ICHD-3 diagnosis, and transient ischemic attack has been excluded	

Reprinted with permission from ICHD [1] ©SAGE

[a]Aphasia is always regarded as a unilateral symptom. Excerpted from the ICHD-3 beta diagnostic criteria for migraine without aura (Code 1.1) and migraine with aura (Code 1.2): Headache Classification Committee of the International Headache Society. ICDH, International Classification of Headache Disorders, Third Edition (ICHD-3)

weakness presents with aura, a diagnosis of hemiplegic migraine is warranted. A variant of hemiplegic migraine, familial hemiplegic migraine, is diagnosed when a first- or second-degree relative also has hemiplegic migraine; in many cases, the causative mutation can be identified by genetic testing.

According to the ICHD-3, diagnosis of CM requires a history of more than 3 months with an average of at least 15 days with headache per month (Table 2.2) [1]. On at least eight of these days, headache must be migrainous in nature; commonly many of the other attacks lack some or all migraine features.

Critical to the diagnosis of both episodic and chronic migraine is that the condition is not clearly attributable to another (secondary) cause, such as head or neck trauma (post-traumatic headache), overuse of acute headache medications (medication overuse headache [MOH]), substance use or medication side effects, or other medical conditions such as vascular disorders (e.g., stroke, subarachnoid hemorrhage, giant cell arteritis), idiopathic intracranial hypertension,

Table 2.2 Diagnostic criteria for chronic migraine (CM)

A. Headache (tension-type-like and/or migraine-like) on ≥15 days per month for >3 months and fulfilling criteria B and C	
B. Occurring in a patient who has had at least five attacks fulfilling criteria B–D for migraine without aura and/or criteria B and C for migraine with aura	
C. On ≥8 days per month for >3 months, fulfilling any of the following:	Criteria C and D for migraine without aura Criteria B and C for migraine with aura Believed by the patient to be migraine at onset and relieved by a triptan or ergot derivative
D. Not better accounted for by another ICHD-3 diagnosis	

Reprinted with permission from International Classification of Headache Disorders [1] ©SAGE intracranial tumors, intracranial or systemic infection (e.g., meningitis, encephalitis, influenza, HIV/AIDS), and disorders of the eyes, nose/sinuses, and mouth/teeth. Medication overuse is the most common cause of headache occurring on 15 or more days per month. MOH diagnostic criteria include:

- Headache occurring on ≥15 days per month in a patient with a preexisting headache disorder.
- Regular overuse for >3 months of one or more drugs that can be taken for acute and/or symptomatic treatment of headache. (Overuse is defined as use of opioids, ergotamine, triptans, combination analgesics, or multiple drug classes ≥10 days per month or use of simple analgesics ≥15 days per month.)
- Not better accounted for by another ICHD diagnosis [1].

Briefly, MOH is characterized by high-frequency headache attacks in conjunction with frequent use of any acute headache agent (prescription or over the counter [OTC]). As a general rule of thumb, MOH is likely in patients with high-frequency headache who use acute headache medications more than 2 days per week on average. The headache attacks in MOH are often not prototypical migraine attacks, as pain is often less severe and bilaterally distributed. In individuals who meet the criteria for both CM and MOH, both disorders should be diagnosed. Treatment of MOH typically requires supervised withdrawal of the overused medication(s) and initiation of appropriate migraine preventive treatment. Overuse is defined as use of opioids, ergotamine, triptans, combination analgesics, or multiple drug classes at least 10 days per month or use of simple analgesics at least 15 days per month [1].

2.2 Headache History

The cornerstone of the clinical evaluation of migraine is the headache history, in which detailed information is gathered about the patient's headache presentation. The headache history should begin with open-ended inquiries about headache symptoms:

- *Tell me about the headaches you've been having.*
- *What symptoms do you typically experience when you have a headache?*
- *How have these headaches interfered with your life or normal activities?*

Open-ended questions help establish rapport with the patient, who often report diagnostic symptoms spontaneously in response. If particular diagnostic criteria are not mentioned, a series of brief closed-ended questions can then be used to assess these features:

- *About how many days per month [or week] do you have headache?*
- *Would you describe the pain in your head as more of a throbbing, pulsing pain or more of a constant tight pressure?*
- *Do you often feel nauseous or sick to your stomach with these headaches?*
- *You mentioned sensitivity to light. Do you experience any sensitivity to normal levels of noise/sound during these attacks?*

The ask-tell-ask method of communication is particularly useful with chronic pain patients as their symptoms are not directly observable: *ask* an open-ended question, *tell* back to them your understanding of their answer, and *ask* if your understanding is correct. This dialogue exchange helps patients feel listened to and understood and be active participants in their treatment. Below is a sample script showing how the ask-tell-ask method can be used with a headache patient:

Clinician: *How would you describe a typical headache attack? (**Ask**)*

Patient: *I know it's coming when I notice that my vision in one eye gets blurry and I start to see colored spots. A little while later I'm doubled over with a terrible throbbing pain in my right temple, and if it's bad enough I might vomit.*

Clinician: *So you often have visual symptoms—we call that an aura—that precedes the pain, and the pain itself has a throbbing quality, usually occurs on one side of your head, and may cause you to vomit.* ***(Tell)***

Clinician: *Am I understanding that correctly or leaving anything out?* ***(Ask)***

Patient: *Yes, it's so bad sometimes I have to leave work and go home to sleep in my bedroom with all the curtains pulled shut.*

Patients with high-frequency headache often have difficulty estimating their attack frequency. Querying the number of days per week *without headache* can also be useful:

Clinician: *On average how many days per month do you have a headache?* ***(Ask)***

Patient: *I'd guess around 20 days a month. I've never really counted before.*

Clinician: *So in a typical week, there's only about 2 days when you are headache-free.* ***(Tell)***

Clinician: *Is that right?* ***(Ask)***

Patient: *Well, maybe I don't have them that often, then. I'd guess it's more like every other day, so about 15 days a month probably.*

Essential information to be gathered from the history includes quantifiable information about the headache attacks (frequency, severity, duration), typical symptoms, and headache-related disability. Frequency of headache should be recorded as days with headache per week or month (not the number of individual headache attacks, as attacks may span multiple days). Headache severity is typically quantified on a 0–10 rating scale in reference to peak pain during an attack, with 0 = no pain and 10 = excruciating pain (or "worst pain imaginable"). Occasionally, a 0–3 rating scale is used in which 0 = no headache, 1 = mild pain, 2 = moderate pain, and 3 = severe pain. However, the 0–3 rating scale is less useful for assessing change over time. Headache duration is quantified as the duration in hours of the attack if left untreated; if the patient falls asleep and then wakes without headache, the duration should be coded as lasting until the patient awoke.

The patient should be queried about typical symptoms accompanying headache in accordance with the ICHD-3 criteria, including pain distribution (unilateral vs. bilateral), quality (pulsatile vs. tight pressure), interference with normal activity, and other features such as nausea, vomiting, photophobia, and phonophobia. The presence of aura has high sensitivity for establishing a migraine diagnosis (i.e., most people with aura have migraine), but because aura occurs among a minority of migraineurs, absence of aura is not indicative of absence of migraine.

Women should be queried as to whether and how often their headaches coincide with menstruation (i.e., ±2 days of onset of menstrual bleeding). Gathering information about initial headache onset, use of acute medications, and recent changes in the headache pattern is helpful for assessing possible secondary causes of headache (post-traumatic headache, medication overuse) and red flags suggestive of a need for neuroimaging (see Sect. 2.5).

2.2.1 Daily Headache Diaries (Self-Monitoring)

The best means of gathering data about recent headache history is through use of a daily headache diary or other self-monitoring form. This is preferable to having patients estimate their past headache activity while in the clinic, which often yields inaccurate information. Paper-and-pencil diaries have been used in headache practice and research for decades (Table 2.3), and more recently, numerous electronic diaries have been developed and adopted. Electronic headache diaries allow for real-time data collection and entry prompts using a smartphone, tablet, or other handheld device. A recent review of available mobile headache diary apps concluded that iHeadache (iOS; Better QOL), ecoHeadache (iOS; ecoTouchMedia), and Headache Diary Pro (Android; Froggyware) were the highest-quality diary apps, though all

TABLE 2.3 Daily headache diary

Day	Monday	Tuesday	Wednesday	Thursday	Friday	Saturday	Sunday
Date	/	/	/	/	/	/	/
Did you have a headache today?	Yes/no	Yes/no	Yes/no	Yes/no	Yes/no	Yes/no	Yes/no
If YES…							
How severe was the pain (from 0 to 10)?	____	____	____	____	____	____	____
What time did it start and end? (duration)	____ to ____ (____ hours)	____ to ____ (____ hours)	____ to ____ (____ hours)	____ to ____ (____ hours)	____ to ____ (____ hours)	____ to ____ (____ hours)	____ to ____ (____ hours)
How disabling was the headache (0=not at all; 10=bed rest required)	____	____	____	____	____	____	____

(continued)

Day	Monday	Tuesday	Wednesday	Thursday	Friday	Saturday	Sunday
Date	/	/	/	/	/	/	/
Symptoms (circle)	Aura Nausea/ vomiting	Aura Nausea/ vomiting	Aura Nausea/ vomiting	Aura Nausea/ vomiting	Aura Nausea/ vomiting	Aura Nausea/ vomiting	Aura Nausea/ vomiting
Treatment/ medications taken							
Relief/ improvement within 2 h?	Yes/no	Yes/no	Yes/no	Yes/no	Yes/no	Yes/no	Yes/no
Possible triggers within previous 24 h? (Stress, poor sleep, missed meal, menstruation, etc.)							

lack published psychometric data [4]. In addition to standard information about headache, some diaries also incorporate entries for variables such as stress, sleep, meals, medication use, and exposure to potential headache triggers. These diaries are a bit more cumbersome for the patient to use but still require only a few minutes each day and afford a wealth of information that can be used by the healthcare provider to monitor headache activity, discern potential headache triggers, and determine the appropriate use of medications.

Regardless of the diary format, patients should record their headache activity and other relevant variables for a period of at least 2 weeks either prior to or immediately following the initial consultation. Monitoring for 4–5 weeks affords capture of all phases of the menstrual cycle. Self-monitoring should occur at least twice daily, spaced throughout the day at regular intervals.

The biggest barrier to self-monitoring is patient nonadherence, which is best prevented by educating the patient as to the importance of regular self-monitoring before she begins. Providers should emphasize the benefits for the patient, including obtaining a comprehensive picture of her headaches, identifying potential triggers, and monitoring treatment efficacy and progress. Pairing monitoring with routine activities (e.g., at meals, bedtime, and/or when taking medications) or using alarm prompts at regular intervals (e.g., every 4 h when awake) may facilitate better adherence. Patients should make diary entries regardless of whether they are having headache at the time of an entry.

2.2.2 *Structured Diagnostic Interviews*

Structured diagnostic interviews are a proven means of establishing a correct migraine diagnosis, as they are standardized and explicitly map onto the ICHD-3 diagnostic criteria. Diagnostic interviews are particularly useful among individuals with complicated presentations or chronic headache subtypes. Some diagnostic interviews may be administered via computer, such as the Structured Diagnostic Interview for Headache (SDIH) [5], the most recent third iteration of which (SDIH-3) corresponds with ICHD-3 [1, 6].

2.3 Headache-Related Disability

Because of migraine's substantial impact on patient functioning, outcomes other than headache characteristics are also of interest. Insofar as migraine interferes with daily functioning, assessment of headache-related disability comprises a vital part of the migraine evaluation and means of assessing response to treatment. Headache-related disability can be easily assessed using one of two measures of headache-related disability, both of which are well-established psychometrically.

The Migraine Disability Assessment (MIDAS) questionnaire [7] is a 7-item measure with 5 questions that inquire about the number of days during the prior 3 months in which headache limited the patient's daily functioning (at work, at school, in household duties, and in leisure activities). Scores range from 0 to 270, and scores >10 indicate that headaches are having a substantial impact on the patient's functioning; scores >20 suggest severe disability. There are two additional questions on the MIDAS concerning average headache frequency and severity, but they are not scored.

The Headache Impact Test (HIT-6) [8] is a 6-item Likert-type questionnaire that inquires about functional impairment, pain severity, and the affective and cognitive effects of headache during the prior 4 weeks. During scoring, each response is transformed using a 6–13 scale. Total scores range from 36 to 78, and scores >55 are indicative of substantial disability and scores >60 of severe disability.

The MIDAS and HIT-6 are intercorrelated ($r = .52$) [9] but quantify disability in different ways: the MIDAS as a function of days of impairment and the HIT-6 as qualitative ratings across broader domains. The MIDAS is more strongly

Table 2.4 Score and interpretation of measures assessing headache-related disability

MIDAS score	Interpretation	HIT-6 score	Interpretation
<5	Minimal disability	<50	Minimal disability
6–10	Mild disability	50–55	Mild disability
11–20	Moderate disability[a]	56–60	Moderate disability[a]
>20	Severe disability[a]	>60	Severe disability[a]

Adapted with permission from Smitherman et al. [6]
HIT-6 Headache Impact Test, *MIDAS* Migraine Disability Assessment questionnaire
[a]Headaches are having a major impact on the patient's functioning; preventive therapy likely indicated

influenced by headache frequency (presumably because it quantifies days of impairment), while the HIT-6 is more influenced by headache severity. When choosing between the two, clinicians should consider their intended purpose and the recall interval desired. The HIT-6 may be more useful if outcome is assessed frequently, as it has a shorter recall interval, although versions of the MIDAS with shorter recall intervals are available (Table 2.4).

2.4 Physical Examination

Because the diagnosis of migraine is made based on self-reported symptoms, physical examination of most migraine patients takes no more than a few minutes and is intended to identify secondary causes of headache. Standard physical examination should include measurement of blood pressure and temperature and more specific evaluation of the head and neck area, including palpation of the scalp and ipsilateral temporal artery and flexion of the neck. Basic neurological examination is essential and should include mental status, testing of cranial nerve responses, and fundoscopic examination [10]. Assessment of motor skills, sensation, and other reflexes is valuable in patients with suspected secondary causes. Observing the patient during the history and components of the physical examination can reveal information about some of these domains (e.g., mental status, coordination, gait). More extensive evaluation is rarely required. Electroencephalogram should not be performed to evaluate headache [11], and neuroimaging is not usually indicated.

2.5 Psychiatric Assessment

In addition to the HIT-6 or MIDAS to assess headache-related disability, screening for comorbid psychiatric symptoms is recommended, particularly for patients with CM or MOH, who present to specialty clinics, or who have been refractory to standard treatments. The 9-item depression module of the Patient Health Questionnaire [12] and Generalized Anxiety Disorder 7-item scale (GAD-7) [13] are recommended for assessing depression and anxiety, respectively. These measures are well validated among medical patients, commonly used in headache settings, and afford extremely brief assessment of core symptoms of these conditions. The GAD-7, though initially developed for identifying GAD specifically, also detects other anxiety disorders [14]. Scores ≥10 on either measure are suggestive of significant psychiatric symptoms and merit more detailed assessment.

Verbal screening for sleep problems can be accomplished with the REST mnemonic, in which the following domains are queried:

- **R**estorative nature of sleep
- **E**xcessive daytime sleepiness
- Frequent/habitual **S**noring
- Perceived adequacy of the patient's average **T**otal sleep time

2.6 Differential Diagnosis

As a general rule, most patients who present for treatment with severe headache attacks that interfere with functioning and that are not temporally related to a head injury have migraine. Symptoms of bilateral pain and a throbbing/pulsatile quality are often present, but many patients have difficulty reporting these symptoms accurately without use of a daily headache diary. The POUND algorithm is a useful tool for differentiating migraine from other headache presentations, as it includes the five features most predictive of migraine [15]:

- **P**ulsating pain quality
- 4–72 h**O**urs duration (if untreated)
- **U**nilateral pain (one sided)
- **N**ausea
- **D**isabling (disrupting daily activities)

Migraine is likely if at least three of the five "POUND" symptoms are present [16]. Given the prevalence of migraine in clinical settings, perhaps the most useful diagnostic skill lies in identifying when a headache disorder is *not* migraine. Tension-type headache (TTH) is the most common headache condition in the world, affecting roughly 50 % of the population annually [17]. Differentiating migraine from TTH is usually rather straightforward, as the presentations are typically opposite to one another (Table 2.5). TTH has a more varied duration (30 min to 7 days), is of lesser intensity, and does not usually interfere with functioning in normal activities. Pain is commonly bilateral and described as having the quality of a tight pressure or band around the scalp. Nausea and vomiting are absent, and photophobia and phonophobia are typically absent as well (though one of photophobia/phonophobia may occur in TTH). Aura does not occur in TTH. Despite its high prevalence, most individuals with TTH do not present for medical care (except those with chronic TTH).

Migraine is also commonly misdiagnosed with cluster headache, sinus headache, and post-traumatic headache.

Cluster headache is quite rare (<0.5 % lifetime prevalence), occurs much more commonly among men than women, and presents as insufferable pain centered around one orbital socket and accompanied by obvious facial swelling, tearing, and redness. Attacks are also of shorter duration (15 min to 3 h) than migraine and occur in clusters, such that sufferers experience multiple attacks within days or weeks interspersed with much longer pain-free periods.

Sinus headache is often diagnosed when patients present with migraine symptoms accompanied by sinus pain/pressure or nasal congestion, when in fact 80 % of these patients meet the criteria for migraine [18]. In the absence of clear signs of acute sinus infection (e.g., purulent discharge, fever), these

Table 2.5 Differential diagnosis: migraine versus tension-type headache (TTH)

Symptom	Migraine	Tension-type headache (TTH)
Criterion B		
Duration	4–72 h	30 min to 7 days
Criterion C (2 of 4 required)		
Pain distribution	Unilateral	Bilateral
Quality	Pulsatile/throbbing	Pressing/tightening
Intensity	Moderate or severe	Mild or moderate
Aggravated by routine activities	Yes	No
Criterion D		
Other features	Nausea, vomiting, *or* both photophobia and phonophobia	No nausea, no vomiting, *and* no more than one of photophobia or phonophobia[a]

[a]Mild nausea may occur in chronic TTH (TTH on ≥15 days per month)

patients likely have migraine triggered or exacerbated by seasonal changes, and migraine should thus be considered as the likely differential diagnosis. Transient ischemic attack and migraine aura both often involve visual disturbances, but in stroke there is typically abrupt onset, visual loss, and other severe neurologic symptoms (e.g., one-sided weakness of the body, loss of balance/coordination, and confusion). Migraine aura, by comparison, develops gradually, is characterized by positive visual symptoms versus visual loss, and is not commonly associated with balance problems or mental confusion.

Many headache disorders resulting from secondary causes have migraine-like presentations in terms of the characteristics of head pain and other symptoms. In instances of secondary headache in which headache onset is clearly linked temporally to another cause, migraine is not diagnosed. (The one exception is chronic headache with migrainous features that occurs in conjunction with regular overuse of acute headache medications, in which case both CM and MOH are diagnosed.) For instance, migrainous headache with onset within 7 days of head/neck trauma is superseded by the diagnosis of post-traumatic headache. Headache presenting as part of other medical conditions (e.g., meningitis, intracranial tumor, HIV) is diagnosed as attributable to those causes. In summary, a migraine diagnosis is warranted when the requisite symptoms are present and when there is no identifiable secondary cause.

2.7 Indications for Neuroimaging

Only a small minority of headache disorders result from underlying intracranial pathology. However, neuroimaging remains frequently overused in headache practice settings, in part stemming from liability concerns and desires to reassure patients that they do not have significant intracranial pathology. Thus, so long as the patient has stable headaches that meet diagnostic criteria for migraine and a normal neurological exam, neuroimaging is not warranted. In such instances, the cost–benefit ratio does not justify imaging, as only 0.9 % of these patients will have evidence of significant intracranial pathology upon imaging [19]. The strength of this recommendation is supported by the American Headache Society's "Choosing Wisely" campaign, which recommends clinicians refrain from performing neuroimaging studies in patients with stable headaches that meet the criteria for migraine [20]. It is recommended to reassure these patients that neuroimaging is not only unwarranted but also very costly with limited yield. In some instances, unwarranted neuroimaging discovers intracranial pathology entirely unrelated to the headache presentation or that is inconsequential. In patients who continue to seek repeated neuroimaging after normal results, this pattern of excessive reassurance seeking suggests underlying psychopathology that merits referral to a mental health provider, coupled with polite but firm refusal to conduct additional tests that are not indicated.

A routine neurological examination is of utmost importance in assessing the need for neuroimaging, as the presence of an abnormal finding on a neurological exam (or altered mental status) should prompt suspicion of intracranial pathology that may warrant imaging. Other signs/symptoms that should raise suspicion of secondary causes are sudden onset (within minutes) of the "worst headache ever" (possible thunderclap headache stemming from subarachnoid hemorrhage, which merits urgent investigation regardless of other features), a notable pattern change of a preexisting headache condition (e.g., dramatic increase in frequency or severity), presence of other systemic symptoms or systemic disease, and new onset of headache in a patient older than 50 years of age [21].

Development of migraine in middle-aged adults is uncommon. In adults over 50 years of age with new-onset headache, giant cell arteritis (i.e., temporal arteritis) should be considered in the differential diagnosis. Giant cell arteritis is characterized by abnormality of the cranial arteries usually evident upon palpation and visual examination in conjunction with erythrocyte sedimentation rate testing. Temporal artery biopsy under local anesthesia is the gold standard for

Table 2.6 SNOOP mnemonic for recognizing headache “red flags”

Systemic disease or symptoms	Chronic medical comorbidity (e.g., history of malignancy, immunocompromised) Fever, chills, significant (and unintentional) weight changes
Neurological signs or symptoms	Abnormal finding on routine neurological exam, altered mental state, seizures
Onset is sudden	“Worst headache of my life” that peaks within minutes[a] First severe headache ever experienced
Onset in a patient over 50 years of age	
Pattern change in headache presentation	Current headache is of different type or much more severe/frequent than prior history

Adapted with permission from Dodick [21]
[a]Requires urgent medical investigation (regardless of other features)

diagnosis of giant cell arteritis, but treatment with corticosteroids and low-dose aspirin is recommended, without waiting for biopsy results, in order to prevent permanent loss of vision [22]. Table 2.6 presents a useful mnemonic (SNOOP) for remembering which signs/symptoms merit further evaluation [21]. Patients with any of these “red flags” should be evaluated more thoroughly for secondary causes, including consideration of neuroimaging if the etiology remains unclear.

When neuroimaging is justified, MRI is generally preferable to computerized tomography (CT) scan because of its superior sensitivity in detecting intracranial causes of headache and lack of radiation exposure [20]. Emergency situations may predicate a justification for using CT instead of MRI, such as an urgent need for imaging in suspected subarachnoid hemorrhage, but otherwise, MRI is the standard of care. Lumbar puncture may be indicated in suspected subarachnoid hemorrhage and other conditions in which it is the accepted standard of care (e.g., meningitis, benign intracranial hypertension).

References

1. Headache Classification Committee of the International Headache Society. The international classification of headache disorders. 3rd ed (beta version). Cephalalgia. 2013;33:629–808.
2. World Health Organization (WHO). International classification of diseases. 10th ed. WHO website. www.who.int/classifications/icd/en/. Accessed 7 Dec 2015.
3. Turner DP, Smitherman TA, Black AK, Penzien DB, Porter JA, Lofland KR, et al. Are migraine and tension-type headache diagnostic types or points on a severity continuum? An exploration of the latent taxometric structure of headache. Pain. 2015;156:1200–7.
4. Hundert AS, Huguet A, McGrath PJ, Stinson JN, Wheaton M. Commercially available mobile phone headache diary apps: a systematic review. JMIR Mhealth Uhealth. 2014;2:e36.
5. Andrew ME, Penzien DB, Rains JC, Knowlton GE, McAnulty RD. Development of a computer application for headache diagnosis: the headache diagnostic system. Int J Biomed Comput. 1992;31:17–24.
6. Smitherman TA, Penzien DB, Rains JC, Nicholson R, Houle TT. Headache. Advances in psychotherapy: evidence-based practice, vol. 30. Cambridge, MA: Hogrefe; 2015.
7. Stewart WF, Lipton RB, Kolodner K, Liberman J, Sawyer J. Reliability of the migraine disability assessment score in a population-based sample of headache sufferers. Cephalalgia. 1999;19:107–14.
8. Kosinski M, Bayliss MS, Bjorner JB, Ware Jr JE, Garber WH, Batenhorst A, et al. A six-item short-form survey for measuring headache impact: the HIT-6. Qual Life Res. 2003;12:963–74.
9. Sauro KM, Rose MS, Becker WJ, Christie SN, Giammarco R, Mackie GF, et al. HIT-6 and MIDAS as measures of headache disability in a headache referral population. Headache. 2010;50:383–95.
10. Donohoe CD. The role of the physical examination in the evaluation of headache. Med Clin N Am. 2013;97:197–216.
11. Langer-Gould AM, Anderson WE, Cohen AB, Cohen AB, Eccher MA, Iverson DJ, et al. The American Academy of Neurology's top five choosing wisely recommendations. Neurology. 2013;81:1004–11.

12. Kroenke K, Spitzer RL, Williams JBW. The PHQ-9: validity of a brief depression severity measure. J Gen Intern Med. 2001;16:606–13.
13. Spitzer RL, Kroenke K, Williams JBW, Lowe B. A brief measure for assessing generalized anxiety disorder: the GAD-7. Arch Intern Med. 2006;166:1092–7.
14. Kroenke K, Spitzer RL, Williams JBW, Monahan PO, Lowe B. Anxiety disorders in primary care: prevalence, impairment, comorbidity, and detection. Ann Intern Med. 2007;146:317–25.
15. Detsky ME, McDonald DR, Baerlocher MO, Tomlinson GA, McCrory DC, Booth CM. Does this patient with headache have a migraine or need neuroimaging? JAMA. 2006;296:1274–83.
16. Michel P, Henry P, Letenneur L, Jogiex M, Corson A, Dartigues JF. Diagnostic screen for assessment of the IHS criteria for migraine by general practitioners. Cephalalgia. 1993;13 Suppl 12:54–9.
17. Stovner LJ, Hagen K, Jensen R, Katsarava Z, Lipton R, Scher A, et al. The global burden of headache: a documentation of headache prevalence and disability worldwide. Cephalalgia. 2007;27:193–210.
18. Schreiber CP, Hutchinson S, Webster CJ, Ames M, Richardson MS, Powers C. Prevalence of migraine in patients with a history of self-reported or physician-diagnosed "sinus" headache. Arch Intern Med. 2004;164:1769–72.
19. Sempere AP, Porta-Etessam J, Medrano V, Garcia-Morales I, Concepción L, Ramos A, et al. Neuroimaging in the evaluation of patients with non-acute headache. Cephalalgia. 2005;25:30–5.
20. Loder E, Weizenbaum E, Frishberg B, Silberstein S. Choosing wisely in headache medicine: the American Headache Society's list of five things physicians and patients should question. Headache. 2013;53:1651–9.
21. Dodick DW. Diagnosing headache: clinical cues and clinical rules. Adv Stud Med. 2003;3:87–92.
22. Smith JH, Swanson JW. Giant cell arteritis. Headache. 2014;54:1273–89.

Chapter 3
Patient Education and Lifestyle Recommendations

3.1 Goals of Treatment

The goals of migraine treatment, both pharmacologic and nonpharmacologic, are to prevent future attacks, reduce headache-related disability, and restore normal functioning as quickly as possible. An in-depth overview of pharmacologic treatments is discussed in Chap. 4, and evidence-based nonpharmacologic treatments are reviewed in Chap. 5. This chapter focuses on education and basic lifestyle recommendations that should be part of all migraine treatment plans.

3.2 Patient Education

As with any other recurrent medical problem, migraine patients should be educated about their condition and their role in managing it to the extent possible. In the United States, for instance, multidisciplinary headache centers hold formal educational sessions, often delivered in a group format, for patients with migraine. Spending time on patient education in the early stages of treatment not only helps patients to be more active participants in their treatment but also facilitates treatment adherence and has positive effects on headache activity and disability [1].

T.A. Smitherman, *Clinician's Manual on Migraine*,
DOI 10.1007/978-3-319-02777-7_3,

TABLE 3.1 Basic components of migraine patient education

Education about migraine	Migraine results from a hypersensitive central nervous system Typical cases of migraine do not warrant neuroimaging or result from brain tumors Migraine is not totally out of patient control—learn ways to better prevent and manage attacks and avoid potential triggers
Education about treatment	The goals of treatment are reduced frequency and improved functioning (permanent resolution of migraine is uncommon) Outcomes are better when adhering to a treatment plan developed with a healthcare provider Honestly discuss concerns about treatment with healthcare provider

Regardless of the intervention, educating the patient about migraine is essential (Table 3.1). Many patients have only cursory knowledge about their own headache disorder, and educating them improves both adherence to treatment and confidence in their own ability to manage aspects of their condition. Migraine is best described to the patient as the result of a hypersensitive central nervous system, in which the patient's nervous system is highly reactive to both internal (physiological changes) and external (environmental, lifestyle) stimuli. For this reason, consistency in behavior is of paramount importance in preventing future headache attacks. Deviations from routine, such as those occurring on the weekends, during holidays, or when traveling, increase vulnerability for experiencing a migraine attack, and patients should be advised to maintain some semblance of structure and routine in these contexts.

The other important aspect of patient education centers on expectations for treatment. Many patients understandably hope that treatment will render them headache-free forever, but usually this is not a realistic goal and only fosters disappointment or excessive treatment-seeking. In fact, in preventive treatment trials, reductions in headache frequency of 50 % or more are considered successful outcomes. Even the most efficacious migraine treatments are not cures, and patients should be encouraged to view meaningful reductions in headache and disability (i.e., improved ability to function in their daily lives) as the primary goals of treatment while realizing that treatment is unlikely to render them completely pain-free.

3.3 Lifestyle Recommendations

In addition to education about migraine and its treatment, all patients should be counseled in basic lifestyle changes of relevance to migraine.

3.3.1 Sleep Management

Because the "migraine brain" is one sensitive to deviations in routine, patients should be counseled on the importance of consistency in sleep and eating habits. Patients should be instructed to obtain 7–9 h of sleep per night (or the amount they require to feel properly rested) and go to bed and get up around the same time every day (even on the weekends). Poor or inadequate sleep appears to be a more common headache trigger than oversleeping, but sleeping in on weekends can perpetuate sleep problems and make it more difficult to rise when workdays resume. Many migraineurs seek bed rest during severe attacks, but they should be instructed to sleep no longer than is necessary for pain relief and to stick to their normal sleep schedule otherwise, as frequent daytime napping can contribute to insomnia at night. Patients with suspected sleep apnea should be referred for comprehensive sleep evaluation via overnight polysomnography, as headache often improves once any underlying sleep disorder is addressed.

Patients with near-daily insomnia, which characterizes the large majority of those with chronic migraine (CM), often warrant a more programmatic sleep intervention from a behavioral health provider. Two randomized controlled trials have shown that a brief behavioral intervention for insomnia improves headache frequency among patients with CM [2, 3]. These interventions involved one or three clinic sessions in which patients were taught strategies to reassociate the bed with sleep, with instructions to practice the strategies every day. Strategies included avoiding activities in bed other than sleep and sex, scheduling a consistent daily sleep schedule, eliminating daytime naps, not eating or drinking close to bedtime, and getting out of bed if unable to fall asleep. Treating and improving insomnia symptoms thus reduce headache attacks, and this treatment option should be considered for those with CM or with frequent insomnia.

3.3.2 Diet

Much has been made about the various food triggers of migraine, but missing meals and fasting are more potent triggers of migraine than particular foods [4], though the pathophysiological mechanisms underlying food triggers remain unclear. Thus, it is far more important that the patient eat meals regularly than initiate an elimination diet in which every conceivable food trigger is avoided [5]. The patient should be instructed in the importance of eating at least three meals daily (i.e., do not skip breakfast) and spaced regularly throughout waking hours. General healthy eating habits should be encouraged: eating balanced healthy meals and limiting consumption of red meat, processed foods, sodium, and sugar. Eating close to bedtime or drinking caffeinated beverages after the early afternoon should be discouraged, although some patients who often awake with morning headache may benefit from eating a late evening snack prior to bed. Alcohol is a common migraine trigger; patients who drink should be cautioned to do so in moderation as dehydration may trigger migraine.

3.3.3 Stress

Stress involves an imbalance between a potential challenge and one's perceived ability to cope with that challenge. Patients typically describe stress as emotional strain resulting from an ongoing major life event or frequent minor hassles. Stress is the most commonly reported trigger of migraine [4], though stress may not precipitate headache immediately upon exposure; attacks are also sometimes precipitated by declines in stress from one day to another (i.e., "let-down" headache) [6]. Despite its relevance, many migraineurs do little to deliberately manage stress. They usually acknowledge stress as a trigger of their attacks but are unaware of why stress perpetuates migraine or else view their stress as uncontrollable.

Educate the patient about the numerous ways in which stress affects migraine, including how stress can predispose a vulnerable individual to developing migraine, promote progression from episodic to chronic migraine, and trigger individual headache attacks. Stress also influences other migraine triggers, such as when high stress is accompanied by poor sleeping and eating habits. Over time, experiencing repeated migraine attacks comes to function as an additional stressor, which maintains sympathetic arousal and further sensitizes the nervous system. Encourage the patient to devote time on a regular basis to stress management: exercise, relaxation training, daily meditation or yoga, or other deliberate activities to promote rest and recovery. Patients with significant life stress or poor coping skills are appropriate candidates for the behavioral therapies discussed in Chap. 5.

3.3.4 Weight Loss

Several studies have demonstrated a link between obesity and migraine among individuals of reproductive age, and this link appears strongest for CM [7]. Obesity appears to be a risk factor for progression of headache frequency over time,

Table 3.2 Lifestyle recommendations for patients with migraine

Lifestyle domain	**Recommendations**
Sleep habits	Keep a consistent sleep schedule (time in bed, time out of bed, even on weekends and when traveling) Try to get between 7 and 9 h of sleep each night Avoid long naps or naps in late afternoon unless necessary for migraine relief Avoid any activities (e.g., watching TV, reading, eating) in the bed other than sleep and sex
Diet	Eat regularly scheduled meals (e.g., three times daily); do not skip meals Maintain a healthy, balanced diet and limit intake of processed foods Drink 64 oz (1.8 L) of water daily Limit or avoid caffeine, especially after early afternoon
Stress management	Exercise regularly (3–4 times a week for at least 30 min) Regularly devote time to stress management activities (relaxation, yoga, meditation, social activities)
Trigger management	Use a headache diary to help identify factors associated with headache onset at least 50 % of the time Be attentive to common triggers such as high stress, menstruation, missing meals, and poor sleep Use "behavioral experiments" to test suspected triggers Avoid triggers that are avoidable, and develop strategies to better manage those that are not
Other	Lose weight if overweight or obese Smoking cessation

presumably through its effects in increasing inflammatory mediators (calcitonin gene-related peptide, adipocitokines) and sympathetic activation [8, 9]. Indirect evidence suggests that weight loss obtained through surgical and behavioral means is associated with reductions in migraine. Patients who are overweight or obese should be counseled to lose weight via diet and exercise [10, 11], and preventive agents with weight loss as a side effect (e.g., topiramate) may be appropriate for obese patients with frequent migraine. Table 3.2 summarizes the major lifestyle recommendations for all patients with migraine.

3.4 Managing Triggers

A routine component of migraine treatment is helping the patient identify and manage triggers of migraine attacks. To the extent that the patient is able to identify reliable triggers, management of these triggers may help to reduce the likelihood of future attacks. In practice, however, accurate identification of headache triggers is challenging, owing to difficulties controlling other triggers, delayed effects of some triggers, and patients failing to notice times in which exposure to a suspected trigger did not precipitate an attack [12].

Identification of headache triggers is aided by the use of a headache diary, on which the patient can record data on the most common triggers of migraine: high stress, menstruation, missing meals, and insufficient sleep. Many paper and electronic headache diaries query these variables. Self-monitoring for a period of several weeks will usually be required, though patients with more frequent attacks (i.e., those with CM) may be able to identify triggers more quickly.

Of interest are those triggers that precede headache within 24 h on 50 % or more of the occasions on which they are encountered. If the potency of a particular trigger is in question, the patient can be instructed in conducting her own "behavioral experiment" in which she deliberately exposes herself to a given trigger on a random day and monitors subsequent headache activity. This should be repeated several days later without exposure to the trigger but while attempting to hold all other variables the same as the first exposure (e.g., daily stress, sleep amount) in order to control for potential interactions between triggers.

Managing triggers that regularly precede migraine can take two forms: avoiding triggers or using problem-solving skills to better manage those that are unavoidable. Avoidance involves the patient eliminating or limiting exposure to triggers by modifying her environment, her behavior, or both. As previously mentioned, eating regular meals, abstaining from particular trigger foods (e.g., red wine, aged cheeses, nuts, caffeine, monosodium glutamate [MSG]), keeping a sufficient and consistent sleep schedule, avoiding bothersome visual or olfactory stimuli (particular lighting, not wearing perfume/cologne), and stopping cigarette smoking are useful avoidance behaviors.

Caffeine triggers headache for some migraineurs, but more commonly caffeine withdrawal is a culprit of headache, even among those who do not consume large quantities of coffee. (Caffeine is included in some over-the-counter combination analgesics taken for migraine, helping to facilitate gastric motility and potentiating analgesia.) For those for whom caffeine is a headache trigger, eliminating caffeine gradually can be beneficial but will usually serve to increase headache activity during the first few days.

Other triggers portend more difficulty to avoid, such as menstruation and weather changes. Women with menstrual migraine may benefit from a constant low-estrogen birth control (i.e., without a week of placebo tablets) or short-term prophylaxis with a longer-acting triptan a couple days before and during menstruation (see Chap. 4). Some women will never or rarely experience another migraine after menopause. Patients who need instruction in developing better stress management skills should be referred to a behavioral provider for formal stress management (see Chap. 5).

References

1. Rothrock JF, Parada VA, Sims C, Key K, Walters NS, Zweifler RM. The impact of intensive patient education on clinical outcome in a clinic-based migraine population. Headache. 2006;46:726–31.
2. Calhoun AH, Ford S. Behavioral sleep modification may revert transformed migraine to episodic migraine. Headache. 2007;47: 1178–83.
3. Smitherman TA, Walters AB, Davis RE, et al. Randomized controlled trial of behavioral insomnia treatment for chronic migraine with comorbid insomnia. Headache. 2016;56:276–91.
4. Kelman L. The triggers or precipitants of the acute migraine attack. Cephalalgia. 2007;27:394–402.
5. Rothrock JF. The truth about triggers. Headache. 2008;3: 499–500.
6. Lipton RB, Buse DC, Hall CB, Tennen H, DeFreitas TA, Borkowski TM, et al. Reduction in perceived stress as a migraine trigger: testing the "let-down headache" hypothesis. Neurology. 2014;82:1395–401.
7. Chai NC, Scher AI, Moghekar A, Bond DS, Peterline BL. Obesity and headache: part I – a systematic review of the epidemiology of obesity and headache. Headache. 2014;54:219–34.
8. Bigal ME, Lipton RB. Modifiable risk factors for migraine progression. Headache. 2006;46:1334–43.
9. Bigal ME, Lipton RB, Holland PR, Goadsby PJ. Obesity, migraine, and chronic migraine: possible mechanisms of interaction. Neurology. 2007;68:1851–61.
10. Bond DS, Vithiananthan S, Nash JM, Thomas JG, Wing RR. Improvement of migraine headaches in severely obese patients after bariatric surgery. Neurology. 2011;76:135–8.
11. Verrotti A, Agostinelli S, D'Egidio C, Di Fonzo A, Carotenuto C, Parisi P, et al. Impact of a weight loss program on migraine in obese adolescents. Eur J Neurol. 2013;20:394–7.
12. Turner DP, Smitherman TA, Martin VT, Penzien DB, Houle TT. Causality and headache triggers. Headache. 2013;53:628–35.

Chapter 4
Pharmacotherapy and Other Medical Treatments

4.1 Introduction

Virtually all of the major treatment options for migraine can be categorized as either acute or preventive in nature. Acute treatments are those used on an as-needed basis and designed to either abort or reduce the severity of a current headache attack. Preventive treatments, by comparison, are typically used on a daily basis and intended to reduce the likelihood of future headache episodes.

4.2 Acute Medications

Acute migraine pharmacotherapy targets a current migraine attack with the aim of returning the patient to normal functioning as soon as possible. Acute treatment can be divided into migraine-specific and nonspecific agents. The migraine-specific agents are those with efficacy for migraine but not other forms of chronic pain. Specific acute migraine agents include the various triptans, ergotamine, and dihydroergotamine (DHE). Nonspecific agents include nonsteroidal anti-inflammatory drugs (NSAIDs), combination analgesics, opioid analgesics, corticosteroids, and antiemetics.

T.A. Smitherman, *Clinician's Manual on Migraine*,
DOI 10.1007/978-3-319-02777-7_4,

4.2.1 Basic Principles of Acute Pharmacotherapy

Virtually all migraine patients should be offered acute pharmacotherapy, including those with very infrequent attacks. These treatments are most effective when used in the developing stages of the migraine attack (within less than an hour of headache onset), versus delaying treatment once pain and other symptoms become severe. Unlike the preventive agents, in which the dosage is started low and gradually increased as needed, acute medications are given more aggressively; these agents are administered at a high effective dose and lowered if there are side effects or safety concerns. In clinical trials of acute migraine pharmacotherapies, the primary outcome of interest usually is the percentage of patients who are pain-free after 2 h. The principles of acute migraine pharmacotherapy include:

- Virtually all patients should be offered acute treatment.
- Overall treatment goal is freedom from pain and returning to functioning within 2 h.
- Use a high effective dose; decrease dose if there are side effects or safety concerns.
- Acute treatments work best if taken within 30–40 min of headache onset.
- Stratify treatment based on the illness severity/disability.
- Limit use of acute medications to no more than 2 days/week.
- Non-oral routes are indicated for patients with vomiting/significant nausea or gastroparesis.
- Avoid prescribing opioids/barbiturates except as a last resort.
- Provide the patient clear instructions on how and when to use the medication.
- At follow-up sessions, query the patient about how she used the medication (normalizing nonadherence helps elicit honest answers).

Acute treatment should be individualized with consideration of the patient's prior drug response, comorbid medical conditions, concurrent medications, and potential for medication overuse. Patients should be cautioned about the role of overusing any acute headache medications (even over-the-counter [OTC] simple analgesics), or combinations of different acute agents, in making headache more frequent over time. Not only does frequent use of acute agents increase headache activity, but it also makes the patient less responsive to triptans. Use of acute agents should be limited to no more than 2 days per week, on average, although up to 3 days per week may be allowed for simple analgesics.

Acute treatment is most effective when stratified by the individual's migraine severity, which may be operationalized as the patient's level of headache-related disability on the Migraine Disability Assessment (MIDAS) questionnaire or Headache Impact Test (HIT-6). Stratified care as a function of illness severity is more efficacious in reducing pain and disability than stepped (escalating) care either across or within attacks, as stepped care can delay optimal treatment [1]. Patients with mild/infrequent disability are appropriate candidates for nonspecific acute treatment, while migraine-specific agents are indicated for those with moderate or severe disability. Triptans represent the standard of care; there is also strong evidence for DHE as an acute treatment if triptans fail [2]. Antiemetics are useful as supplementary treatment when vomiting or severe nausea is present. Parenteral routes are recommended for patients with vomiting/significant nausea or to confer more rapid symptom relief among those with allodynia.

Improper adherence to acute medications is a leading cause of failed acute therapy, much of which stems from poor patient–provider communication. Educate the patient about the rationale for selecting a given agent and provide clear instructions regarding limits on frequency of use and appropriate timing of taking the medication. If a patient reports inadequate response to an acute agent, before altering the treatment plan, she should be queried as to whether she used the medication properly. A common reason for poor response is waiting too late in the headache episode to administer the medication, at which point triptans have limited efficacy because central sensitization has already manifested within the attack. For this reason, patients should be discouraged from waiting to determine if a developing headache will progress to a migraine. Instead, they should be instructed to take the acute agent when pain is mild.

The goal for acute treatment is freedom from pain and a return to functioning within 2 h. "Rescue" or backup medications are used in the event that acute treatment fails. Rescue agents may not completely eliminate pain, but they provide some relief and can help avoid an emergency hospital visit. Injectable sumatriptan and DHE, as well as parenteral NSAIDs, are common rescue medications; dopamine antagonists are used if vomiting or severe nausea remains. However, neither triptans nor ergots should be used as recue medications for each other, as they interact. If the patient responds to the initial triptan but headache recurs within 24 h, a second dose is often effective in treating recurrence. Table 4.1 denotes the proven efficacious acute medications for migraine as reported in a recent evidence-based assessment by the American Headache Society [2].

4.2.2 Triptans

Triptans, selective serotonin ($5HT_{1B/1D}$) agonists, are the only class of drug specifically developed to treat migraine, and their selectivity in targeting migraine pathophysiology is superior to other agents. Sumatriptan was the first to be developed and was released under the brand name Imitrex in the early 1990s. Subsequently numerous other triptans were developed by other pharmaceutical companies: naratriptan, zolmitriptan, rizatriptan, almotriptan, eletriptan, and frovatriptan. Sumatriptan is also available in a combination formulation with naproxen, which confers greater rates of sustained 24 h pain freedom than sumatriptan alone but is

TABLE 4.1 Efficacious acute medications for migraine in adults (with typical single dose)

Strong (level A) evidence	
Drug class	**Migraine-specific medications (dose)**
Triptans[a]	Almotriptan (12.5 mg) Eletriptan (20 mg, 40 mg, 80 mg) Frovatriptan (2.5 mg) Naratriptan (1 mg, 2.5 mg) Rizatriptan (5 mg, 10 mg) Zolmitriptan (2.5 mg, 5 mg; nasal spray 2.5 mg, 5 mg) Sumatriptan (25 mg, 50 mg, 100 mg; nasal spray 10 mg, 20 mg; transdermal patch 6.5 mg; SC 4 mg, 6 mg) Sumatriptan/naproxen (85/500 mg)
Ergot alkaloids/ derivatives	Dihydroergotamine[a] (DHE; nasal spray 2 mg; inhaler 1 mg)
	Nonspecific medications (dose)
NSAIDs	Aspirin (500 mg) Ibuprofen (200 mg, 400 mg) Naproxen (500 mg, 550 mg) Diclofenac[a] (50 mg, 100 mg)
Combination analgesic	Acetaminophen/aspirin/caffeine (500/500/130 mg)
Opioid analgesic	Butorphanol (nasal spray 1 mg)
Simple analgesic	Acetaminophen 1000 mg (for non-debilitating attacks not requiring bed rest)
Moderate (level B) evidence	
Ergot alkaloids/ derivatives	DHE (IV, IM, SC 1 mg) Ergotamine /caffeine[a] (1/100 mg)
NSAIDs	Flurbiprofen (100 mg) Ketoprofen (100 mg) Ketorolac (IV/IM 30–60 mg)

(continued)

TABLE 4.1 (continued)

Antiemetics (dopamine antagonists)	Chlorpromazine (IV 12.5 mg) Droperidol (IV 2.75 mg) Metoclopramide (IV 10 mg) Prochlorperazine (IV/IM 10 mg; PR 25 mg)
Opioid analgesics	Codeine/acetaminophen (25/400 mg) Tramadol/acetaminophen (75/650 mg)
Other	$MgSO_4$ for migraine with aura (1–2 g) Isometheptene (65 mg)

Adapted from Marmura et al. [2] ©American Headache Society
[a]FDA approved for acute treatment of migraine in adults. Note: almotriptan (recommended dose 6.25 or 12.5 mg), sumatriptan/naproxen (recommended dose 10/60 mg), and zolmitriptan nasal spray (recommended dose 2.5 mg) has FDA approval for adolescents 12+ years of age; rizatriptan (recommended dose 5 mg or 10 mg) is FDA approved for children 6–17 years of age. In the United States, over-the-counter drugs with FDA approval for adults include Excedrin® Migraine (aspirin + acetaminophen + caffeine), Advil® Migraine (ibuprofen), and Motrin® Migraine Pain (ibuprofen). *DHE* dihydroergotamine. Provided dose is for oral tablet unless route of administration otherwise denoted. *SC* subcutaneous, *IV* intravenous, *IM* intramuscular, *PR* suppository

not yet available in generic form and thus costly for many patients. (As a result many providers instead prescribe both generic sumatriptan and naproxen to be taken simultaneously, for patients with long-lasting attacks.) The triptans presumably are efficacious as a result of their action in constricting cerebral blood vessels and reducing nociception in trigeminovascular pain pathways.

Speed of onset and route of administration are usually the most important determinants in selecting a triptan. All triptans are available in tablet form; sumatriptan has the widest range of available formulations. Non-oral preparations (injection, nasal spray, transdermal patch, suppository) should be the first choice for patients with severe nausea or any vomiting and considered for patients with poor gastric motility (i.e., gastroparesis). These parenteral routes of administration confer more rapid onset as they do not have to first pass through the stomach. Intranasal acute treatments should be done with the head upright, and the patient should not attempt to sniff the medicine down the nose or tip the head back, as this reduces efficacy.

Though the triptans share more commonalities than differences, a recent meta-analysis quantified the relative efficacy of the various triptan oral tablet formulations across 74 randomized trials [3]. The primary endpoints were pain-free response at 2 h and sustained pain-free response at 24 h, expressed in odds ratios (ORs) of triptan versus placebo. All triptans outperformed placebo and most were 2–4 times more likely to yield pain-free responses at the endpoints (Fig. 4.1) [3]. As compared to one another, at the 2 h time point, eletriptan 40 mg was superior to sumatriptan 50 mg, almotriptan 2.5 mg, zolmitriptan 12.5 mg, and naratriptan 2.5 mg (ORs 1.5–2.9 for pain freedom vs. the other triptans). Rizatriptan and zolmitriptan had the next best efficacy at 2 h. Eletriptan 40 mg was also superior to sumatriptan 50 mg, rizatriptan 10 mg, and naratriptan 2.5 mg on pain freedom at 24 h (ORs ranged from 1.6 to 1.8) [3].

Thus, although eletriptan is most likely to yield a pain-free response at either time point, all triptans are superior to placebo, and rizatriptan and zolmitriptan also produced comparatively favorable pain-free responses [3]. Frovatriptan and naratriptan have somewhat lower efficacy but are longer-lasting (particularly frovatriptan, which has a 26 h half-life) and thus often used for menstrual migraine prevention or attacks typically lasting >24 h. As this review only assessed oral formulations, comparisons with non-oral routes of administration cannot be made, though another recent meta-analysis concluded that alternative routes of administration (injection, orally disintegrating tablet) compare favorably to standard oral tablets [4].

The majority of patients experience pain relief 2 h after a standard dose of triptan [4]. A patient who does not respond

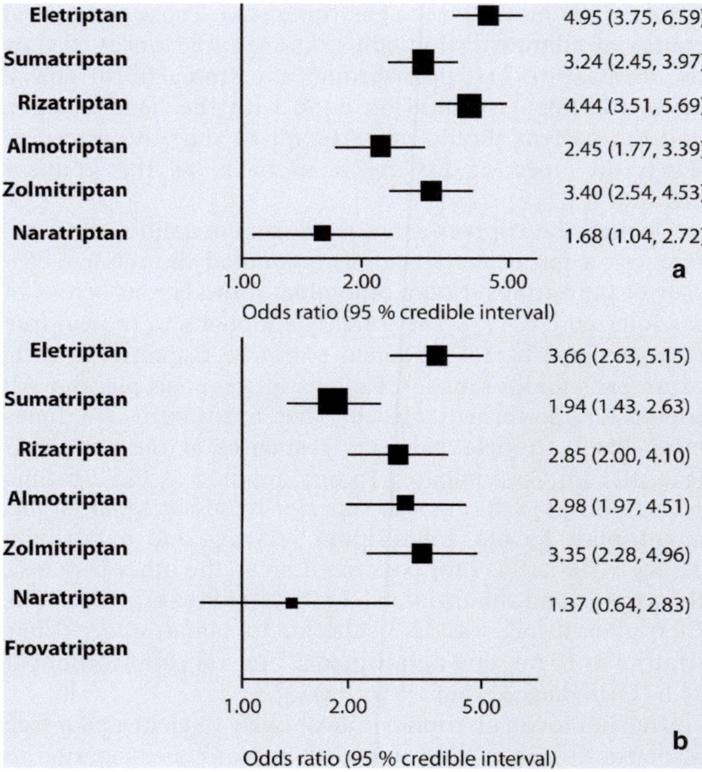

FIG. 4.1 Forest plot of the primary multiple treatment comparison meta-analysis results, triptans versus placebo. (**a**) Pain-free response at 2 h; (**b**) 24 h sustained pain-free response (Reproduced with permission from Thorlund et al. [3] ©SAGE)

to one triptan usually should be tried on at least one other triptan, or using different route of administration, before resorting to another class of acute medication, as the large majority of migraine patients will respond to at least one triptan. As mentioned earlier, patients with a brief or incomplete response to sumatriptan can take naproxen simultaneously with sumatriptan, which often promotes a more long-lasting or complete response.

Triptans are relatively safe, but because of their vasoactive properties, they are contraindicated in patients with cardiovascular disease and related conditions (e.g., obesity, uncontrolled hypertension, severe liver disease). Possibility of serotonin syndrome must be considered among patients taking a triptan and another serotonin agonist, although the risk of serotonin syndrome from taking a triptan and a newer antidepressant (SSRI or SNRI) appears incredibly low, in large part because these agents act on different serotonin receptor subtypes [5].

4.2.3 Ergotamine Derivatives

Ergotamine tartrate and DHE are migraine-specific agents that are serotonin agonists with vasoconstrictive effects. DHE has poor oral bioavailability but has strong evidence for acute migraine treatment in intranasal form. Rhinitis is a common side effect of intranasal DHE. DHE injection and ergotamine/caffeine tablets have moderate efficacy for migraine [2]. Efficacy for ergot alkaloids is thus not as strong as for the triptans [4] and side effects are more significant; ergotamine derivatives are generally used in patients with severe migraines that have not responded to adequate triptan therapy.

Nausea and vomiting are common side effects, particularly of intravenous DHE, which can be reduced by intramuscular injection instead or by adding an antiemetic. Contraindications include vascular conditions (e.g., heart disease, coronary artery vasospasm, uncontrolled hypertension) as well as renal or hepatic failure, pregnancy, and in patients using potent CYP3A4 enzyme inhibitors (e.g., protease inhibitors, macrolide antibiotics such as erythromycin). Life-threatening peripheral ischemia is associated with use of ergot alkaloids and CYP3A4 inhibitors. Ergotamine, DHE, and triptans should not be taken within 24 h of one another.

4.2.4 Nonsteroidal Anti-inflammatory Drugs and Combination Analgesics

For infrequent migraine attacks that are not severe or that evolve slowly, NSAIDs and combinations represent a reasonable first-line treatment. The most common side effects of NSAIDs are gastrointestinal in nature (bloating, dyspepsia, ulcers, gastrointestinal bleeding), which can often be relieved by taking with food. In some patients NSAIDs raise blood pressure, and they can interfere with the efficacy of antihypertensive drugs.

The most commonly used OTC combination analgesic is acetaminophen–aspirin–caffeine (500 mg/500 mg/130 mg). Caffeine potentiates the analgesic effects of the other compounds, promotes gastric motility, and has vasoconstrictive effects. In addition to elevating risk for medication overuse headache (MOH), frequent use of caffeine-containing combination analgesics can cause caffeine withdrawal headaches, tachycardia, and insomnia.

4.2.5 Opioid Analgesics and Butalbital

Both the American Academy of Neurology and American Headache Society recommend against use of opioids or butalbital for treating migraine except among patients who have not responded to other interventions [6, 7]. These medications are not as effective for migraine or migraine disability as the migraine-specific agents and portend the greatest risks for both dependency/abuse and progression to chronic headache (CM) or MOH [8].

Common side effects include sedation, cognitive slowing, dizziness, nausea, and constipation. Patients who claim that opioids do not produce these side effects and are the only medication that reduces their migraine are likely showing tolerance from overuse or demonstrating drug-seeking behavior. Patients with any history of substance use problems should not be prescribed opioids nor should patients on an MAOI antidepressant.

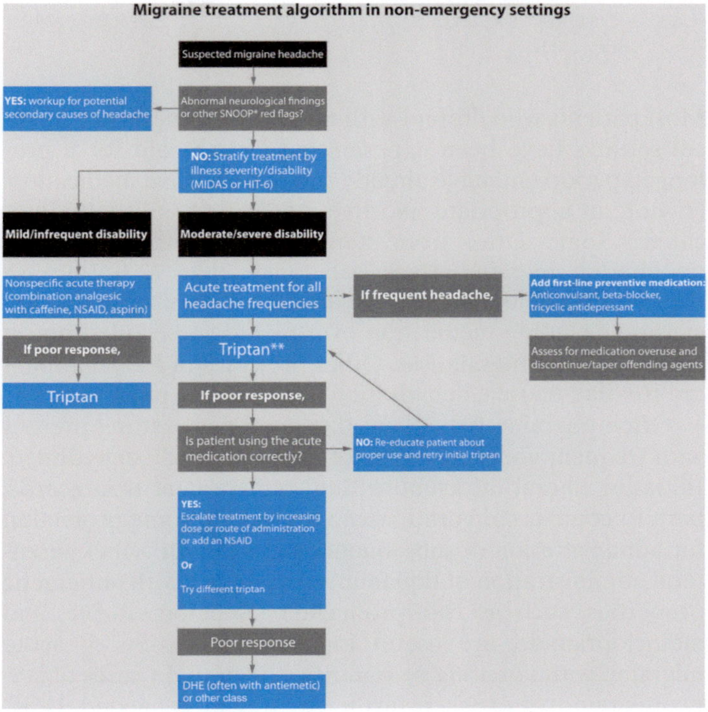

FIG. 4.2 Migraine treatment algorithm in nonemergency settings. *DHE* dihydroergotamine, *NSAID* nonsteroidal anti-inflammatory drugs. **SNOOP* **S**ystemic disease or symptoms, **N**eurological signs or symptoms, **O**nset is sudden, **O**nset in a patient over 50 years of age, **P**attern change in headache presentation; **For vomiting and severe nausea, consider adding an antiemetic or using parenteral administration

4.2.6 Acetaminophen

The evidence for acetaminophen is not as strong as that for the NSAIDs or combination analgesics, and thus, acetaminophen is not recommended as a first-line agent. A summary of migraine treatments in nonemergency settings is seen in Fig. 4.2.

4.2.7 Acute Treatment of Migraine in Emergency Settings

Most patients who present with migraine in emergency medical settings have been experiencing severe pain for a prolonged period and have already tried an abortive medication. (If not, an appropriate abortive medication is usually indicated.) Some suffer from status migrainosus, in which a debilitating migraine attack lasts longer than 72 h. Because the severity and duration of the attack are atypical, secondary causes (including medication overuse) must be ruled out in cases of status migrainosus. Other priorities of ER treatment are treating nausea, dehydration, and residual pain.

Often migraine patients in the emergency setting present with frequent vomiting or are otherwise already dehydrated. Initiating liberal intravenous fluid replacement is indicated, both to combat dehydration and to provide some protection for administration of subsequent agents [9]. Off-label parenteral administration of dopamine antagonists with antiemetic properties, such as chlorpromazine, prochlorperazine, and metoclopramide, are useful for rapid reduction of acute migraine with vomiting or significant nausea. In cases of status migrainosus or when further treatment is needed, DHE and subcutaneous sumatriptan are efficacious treatment options, followed by parenteral NSAIDs [9]. Patients unresponsive to this combination may require hospitalization to undergo repeated intravenous DHE.

Opioids should not be used as first-line agents even in most emergency settings, as these agents are less efficacious as and interfere with other acute medications, have significant side effects, and portend increased risk for repeated emergency hospital visits and development of MOH. Strikingly, many physicians in emergency hospital settings continue to dispense opioids to migraineurs on a routine basis [10]. Patients presenting to emergency hospital settings should be provided a referral to a neurologist with expertise in headache for regular continued care and detailed evaluation of their headache problem.

4.3 Preventive Medications

Preventive agents are those taken regularly, usually daily, to prevent future headache attacks. The most well-established medications for migraine prevention are tricyclic antidepressants, beta-blockers, and antiepileptics, each of which was developed to treat a condition other than migraine. Discovery of their utility in migraine was largely serendipitous, but numerous clinical trials have confirmed their efficacy for migraine prevention.

4.3.1 Basic Principles of Preventive Pharmacotherapy

Preventive pharmacotherapy is indicated for migraine sufferers with 6 or more headache days per month or who have at least 3 headache days per month with significant functional impairment (rule of thumb: one migraine/week merits consideration for preventive therapy). Preventive treatment may be considered in patients who fall shy of these thresholds but are not indicated for those with ≤3 headache days/month without impairment or those with only one headache/day per month regardless of impairment [11]. These recommendations come from the American Migraine Prevalence and Prevention (AMPP) Advisory Group and were developed for epidemiologic research, and thus clinical considerations may dictate alteration in some cases.

All patients requiring preventive treatment should also be provided acute treatment, usually with triptans if appropriate, with clear limits on frequency of their use. Those requiring preventive treatment should be queried carefully about their current use of any acute agents (including OTC medications), as ongoing medication overuse will limit their responsiveness to preventive pharmacotherapy and likely require supervised withdrawal from the offending medication before efficacy with a preventive agent can be obtained. Preventive pharmacotherapies are not a recognized cause of MOH.

The primary determinants of selecting a preventive medication are based on efficacy for migraine, potential side effects and drug interactions, and comorbid medical conditions. The chosen preventive drug should be started slowly and titrated up to the lowest efficacious dose ("start low, go slow"). Most preventive agents require an adequate trial of 2–3 months to assess treatment response, during which time the patient can monitor headache activity and medication use in a headache diary. Full effect may not be evident for as long as 6 months. Patients should be advised not to stop taking the medication if their headaches begin to improve, as this is a common cause of relapse. If the patient has a sustained strong response, considering discontinuing or tapering the medication may be appropriate. The principles of preventive migraine pharmacotherapy include:

- Treatment goal are reduction in attack frequency (≥50 %) and disability.
- Indicated for those with 3 or more headache days/month with impairment (or 6 or more days without impairment).
- Start dosage low and increase slowly if warranted ("start low, go slow").
- Treatment response may not be evident for several months.
- Caution the patient not to stop taking the medication if headaches improve.
- Instruct patient to use a headache diary to monitor efficacy.
- Consider tapering/discontinuing preventive medication if migraine is well controlled after 6 months.
- Separate agent will often be required to treat comorbid conditions.

In preventive trials, the main outcome of interest is proportion of patients with ≥50 % reduction in frequency of headache attacks. In clinical settings, reductions in headache frequency and headache-related disability are primary outcomes, though reductions in headache severity, headache duration, and decreased usage of or increased responsiveness to acute medications are also of importance.

Although ideally one drug could be used to treat both migraine and a particular comorbid medical condition (e.g., depression, anxiety), in practice this is often unsuccessful. The dosage required for treating migraine is often much different than that needed to adequately treat the comorbidity. In cases of comorbid conditions, often multiple agents are required, each selected based on its efficacy for the individual condition and with attention to potential drug interactions.

Table 4.2 denotes the efficacious preventive treatments for episodic migraine (EM) in adults, as reported in the preventive treatment guidelines developed jointly by the American Academy of Neurology and the American Headache Society [12, 13].

4.3.2 Tricyclics

Amitriptyline in particular has a long history of use for migraine prophylaxis and was until recently considered a first-line agent. Amitriptyline is efficacious for migraine prevention but was downgraded to a second-line treatment in the most recent preventive treatment guidelines, in light of the fact that existing studies on amitriptyline were marked by high rates of dropouts (≥20 %). Adverse anticholinergic and antihistaminic effects, including sedation and weight gain, can limit tolerability, but amitriptyline may be particularly useful for migraineurs who have difficulty sleeping so long as it is given at bedtime. The dosage required for treating migraine is far less than that used for depression, and at those higher doses, side effects become particularly pronounced. Tricyclics can also lower seizure threshold and may not be appropriate for elderly patients or those with significant suicidal ideation given its toxicity in overdose. Comparison studies with the established anticonvulsants suggest that amitriptyline has similar efficacy.

Table 4.2 Efficacious preventive medications for episodic migraine in adults (with usual therapeutic dose per day)

Strong (level A) evidence	
Drug class	
Antiepileptics	Divalproex sodium[a]/sodium valproate[a] (500–1500 mg) Topiramate[a] (50–200 mg)
Beta-blockers	Propranolol (40–240 mg) Metoprolol (50–200 mg) Timolol (10–30 mg)
Triptans (for short-term prevention of menstrual migraine only)	Frovatriptan (2.5 mg QD or BID)
Nonprescription	Petasites (butterbur extract; 50–75 mg BID)[b]
Moderate (level B) evidence	
Antidepressants	Amitriptyline[c] (25–150 mg) Venlafaxine 150 mg
Beta-blockers	Atenolol (50–200 mg) Nadolol (20–160 mg)
Triptans (for short-term prevention of menstrual migraine only)	Naratriptan (1 mg BID) Zolmitriptan (2.5 mg BID or TID)
Other	NSAIDs (fenoprofen, ibuprofen, ketoprofen, naproxen, naproxen sodium) Magnesium (400–600 mg) MIG-99 (feverfew CO2-extract) Riboflavin (400 mg) Histamine (subcutaneous; 1–10 ng N-alpha-methyl histamine 2 times/week)

Adapted from Silberstein et al. [12] and Holland et al. [13]

[a]FDA approved for migraine in adults; topiramate has FDA approval for adolescents 12–17 years of age

[b]Significant safety concerns (see Sect. 4.3.5)

[c]Amitriptyline is efficacious and widely used for migraine prevention, but its evidence rating was downgraded because prior trials had high rates of treatment attrition ($\geq$20 %)

4.3.3 Beta-Blockers

Propranolol is well established for migraine prevention, and recently metoprolol was also judged to be efficacious. Common side effects include drowsiness, sleep problems, weight gain, and fatigue.

4.3.4 Antiepileptics

Topiramate, sodium valproate, and divalproex sodium are each well established for prophylaxis of EM. Topiramate also has efficacy for CM as established in multiple clinical trials, including patients with CM who also have medication overuse. Cognitive impairment is a common adverse effect, as are sleepiness, nausea, and paresthesia. Unlike valproate and divalproex, which often cause weight gain, topiramate is associated with weight loss. These agents are contraindicated in patients with hepatic dysfunction and kidney stones or who are pregnant or planning to become pregnant; antiepileptics can worsen comorbid depression in some patients. Periodic monitoring of blood levels is recommended given risks of liver damage and pancreatitis and to pregnant women [12].

4.3.5 Nonprescription Preventive Medications

The extract of the butterbur plant (*Petasites*) has evidence of efficacy for EM from multiple trials [13]; longer studies are needed to assess its long-term effects. Gastrointestinal side effects are not uncommon. Careful preparation is required to remove toxic alkaloids in butterbur extract, and thus hepatic toxicity is a major safety concern as butterbur preparations are not actively regulated by any governing agency. Many NSAIDs effectively prevent migraine, but the effects are rather modest; the more well-established preventive medications are better treatment options for most patients.

4.3.6 Prevention of Menstrually Related Migraine

Though they are commonly used as acute agents, administration of particular triptans (e.g., frovatriptan, naratriptan, or zolmitriptan) prior to and during menstruation is efficacious for preventing menstrually related migraine attacks. The triptan is usually taken for 5–6 days, beginning 2 days prior to menses; most trials have used twice-daily dosing. Because menstrual migraine is triggered by drops in estrogen, continuous low-dose estrogen contraception is another preventive treatment option.

4.3.7 Botulinum Toxin for Prevention of Chronic Migraine

Botulinum toxin A has approval by the Food and Drug Administration (FDA) in the United States, Canada, and United Kingdom for prevention of chronic, but not episodic, migraine. Botulinum in small doses promotes muscular relaxation via acetylcholine inhibition and also has analgesic properties. The utility of botulinum for migraine was discovered when patients receiving injections for cosmetic purposes later reported reductions in headache. Botulinum has demonstrated superiority to placebo injections in multiple randomized clinical trials, although a meta-analysis concluded outcomes were rather modest (2.3 fewer headache days/month vs. placebo injection) and not superior to established preventive medications for EM (e.g., amitriptyline, antiepileptics) [14]. Many patients have difficulty obtaining botulinum treatment because it is expensive and typically requires insurance pre-authorization as well as repeated dosing over time.

The injection protocol was established in a series of trials from the Phase III REsearch Evaluating Migraine Prophylaxis Therapy (PREEMPT) program. Dosage is 155 units divided equally among 31 fixed head/neck sites

(5 units/site): frontalis, corrugator, procerus, occipitalis, temporalis, trapezius, and cervical paraspinal muscle groups. A detailed description of the PREEMPT injection paradigm is seen in Table 4.3 [15].

Because effects taper over time, injections are often repeated in 3+ month intervals and may be gradually spaced further apart to see if continued injections are needed. Side effects are generally mild and temporary and include neck pain, eyelid drooping, and facial muscle paralysis/spasm. Botulinum is contraindicated in children and adolescents, pregnant women, and those with an infection at one or more injection sites. Extreme caution should be used when considering botulinum for patients with neuromuscular diseases or taking drugs that affect neuromuscular transmission.

Table 4.3 The PREEMPT study injection paradigm

Head/neck area	**Recommended dose: total dosage and number of sites**[a]
Frontalis[b]	20 units in 4 sites
Corrugator[b]	10 units in 2 sites
Procerus	5 units in 1 site
Occipitalis[b]	30 units in 6 sites, rebreak up to 40 units in 8 sites
Temporalis[b]	40 units in 8 sites, rebreak up to 50 units in 10 cites
Trapezius	30 units in 6 sites, rebreak up to 50 units in 10 sites
Cervical paraspinal muscle group	20 units in 4 sites
Total dose range	155 units to 195 units

Reproduced with permission from Blumenfeld et al. [15] ©Wiley

[a]Each intramuscular site = 0.1 mL = 5 U onabotulinumtoxinA

[b]Dose distributed bilaterally for the minimum 155 U dose

4.3.8 Calcitonin Gene-Related Peptide Agents

Calcitonin gene-related peptide (CGRP) is a neuropeptide that causes vasodilation and neurogenic inflammation when released at trigeminal nuclei, and its role in migraine pathophysiology has been recognized for many years [16]. Despite promising early results as an acute treatment, efforts to develop the CGRP antagonist telcagepant as a migraine preventive were abandoned after 2.5 % of patients taking telcagepant developed liver aminotransferase elevations orders of magnitude above normal [17]. Development of other CGRP antagonists has stalled somewhat out of concerns about liver damage or limited oral bioavailability, though these drugs appear to have more favorable cardiovascular effect profiles than the triptans as they appear less likely to cause vasoconstrictor-related adverse effects [16].

The newest wave of CGRP efforts centers on developing monoclonal antibodies to CGRP and its receptors, the long half-lives of which allow monthly intravenous instead of daily dosing. These agents thus have potential as migraine preventives with less risk of hepatic toxicity. Recent phase II trials among patients with EM show that these agents reduce migraine frequency approximately 1 day per month more than placebo; common adverse events include pain, erythema, and respiratory tract infections [18, 19]. Despite promising early trials, larger phase III trials are needed to assess longer-term effects and safety over time. CGRP represents the most-researched target for migraine drug development at present, and there is optimism among some headache specialists that these drugs may become the next major breakthrough in migraine since the triptans, though none are yet available commercially.

4.3.9 Ineffective Preventive Medications

The selective serotonin reuptake inhibitors (SSRIs) are not efficacious for migraine prevention [20], and only one serotonin/norepinephrine reuptake inhibitor (SNRI), venlafaxine, has moderate efficacy based on small trials [12]; it is not preferred to the more established preventive agents but may be a useful option for certain patients. Lamotrigine is not effective and clomipramine is probably ineffective.

Despite early positive reports, gabapentin (at any dose) is not effective for migraine prophylaxis, as concluded by a recent Cochrane review, which included negative findings on gabapentin that previously may have been suppressed or misrepresented [21].

4.4 Other Medical Therapies

4.4.1 Electrical and Magnetic Neuromodulation

The field of headache is witnessing a growth of interest in neuromodulation. Cefaly® (Herstal, Belgium), a supraorbital transcutaneous electric nerve stimulation (TENS) device, is the first TENS unit to receive FDA approval for migraine prevention. The device requires a prescription and is worn attached to the forehead via a band containing self-adhesive electrodes. A mild electric current is used to stimulate the trigeminal nerve, and the unit is to be used for 20 min daily. Common side effects include discomfort wearing the device, sedation/sleepiness, and headache after treatment. Most existing studies are small but have shown favorable results in comparison to sham stimulation, although the study methodologies and outcomes are generally not as strong as those with the well-established preventive pharmacotherapies.

Interest is also growing in transcranial magnetic stimulation (TMS) for both acute and preventive treatment of migraine. One sham-controlled trial demonstrated efficacy for acute treatment of migraine with aura [22]. TMS appears safe and may be a useful alternative to more traditional pharmacotherapies or established behavioral interventions [23], but more large controlled trials are needed to establish its efficacy.

4.4.2 Interventional Procedures

Many headache practitioners report positive results with peripheral nerve blocks (commonly of the greater occipital nerve) and trigger point injections for high-frequency headache disorders (CM, chronic tension-type headache) and occipital neuralgia. Both procedures are typically conducted with a local anesthetic (commonly lidocaine or bupivacaine), and corticosteroids are sometimes combined with anesthetic in peripheral nerve blocks. Pain, numbness, and light-headedness are common adverse effects, but these procedures generally appear to be rather safe and well tolerated. Despite their frequent use in clinical settings, there are no accepted guidelines for dosing, injection sites, or injection schedules, and few well-controlled prospective trials have examined the efficacy of these procedures [24].

Owing in large part to their efficacy in cluster headache, interventional procedures targeting the occipital nerves or sphenopalatine ganglion (SPG) are a current source of much current migraine research. Occipital nerve stimulation via implantable pulse generators has some evidence of efficacy for CM from multiple controlled trials, but the effects on headache are somewhat modest when compared to sham stimulation (2.6 fewer headache days/month), owing to large placebo response rates [25]. Common adverse effects are persistent implant site pain, infection, and lead migration, the latter of which not uncommonly requires surgical intervention. Similarly, small trials of SPG nerve blocks or electric stimulation have shown some promise, but a need for larger trials precludes recommendation as a routine intervention. Several small open-label studies have produced mixed findings for the efficacy of vagus nerve stimulation, and like most of the other "emerging therapies" reviewed in this section, large controlled trials are lacking.

4.4.3 Surgical Treatment

Surgical treatments for migraine currently lack evidence of efficacy [26]. In part, this limited efficacy stems from the large variety of surgical sites targeted and procedures employed, as well as limited data on the long-term effects of these invasive procedures. As such, the American Headache Society explicitly recommends against surgical attempts to "deactivate" migraine trigger sites for any form of migraine [7]. Conflicting results have emerged regarding a potential link between patent foramen ovale (PFO) and migraine, and the evidence that PFO closure improves migraine is weak [27].

References

1. Lipton RB, Stewart WF, Stone AM, Láinez MJA, Sawyer JPC. Stratified care versus step care strategies for migraine. The Disability in Strategies of Care Study: a randomized trial. JAMA. 2000;284:2599–605.
2. Marmura MJ, Silberstein SD, Schwedt TJ. The acute treatment of migraine in adults: The American Headache Society evidence assessment of migraine pharmacotherapies. Headache. 2015;55:3–20.
3. Thorlund K, Mills EJ, Wing P, Ramos E, Chatterjee A, Druyts E, et al. Comparative efficacy of triptans for the abortive treatment of migraine: a multiple treatment comparison meta-analysis. Cephalalgia. 2014;34:258–67.
4. Cameron C, Kelly S, Hsieh SC, Murphy M, Chen L, Kotb A, et al. Triptans in the acute treatment of migraine: a systematic review and network meta-analysis. Headache. 2015;55:221–35.
5. Evans RW, Tepper SJ, Shapiro RE, Sun-Edelstein C, Tietjen GE. The FDA alert on serotonin syndrome with use of triptans combined with selective serotonin reuptake inhibitors or selective serotonin-norepinephrine reuptake inhibitors: American Headache Society position paper. Headache. 2010;50:1089–99.
6. Langer-Gould AM, Anderson WE, Cohen AB, Eccher MA, Iverson DJ, Potrebic SB, et al. The American Academy of Neurology's top five choosing wisely recommendations. Neurology. 2013;81:1004–11.
7. Loder E, Weizenbaum E, Frishberg B, Silberstein S. Choosing wisely in headache medicine: The American Headache Society's list of five things physicians and patients should question. Headache. 2013;53:1651–9.

8. Bigal ME, Serrano D, Buse D, Scher A, Stewart WF, Lipton RB. Acute migraine medications and evolution from episodic to chronic migraine: a longitudinal population-based study. Headache. 2008;48:1157–68.
9. Gelfand AA, Goadsby PJ. A neurologist's guide to acute migraine therapy in the emergency room. Neurohospitalist. 2012;2:51–9.
10. Friedman BW, West J, Vinson DR, Minen MT, Restivo A, Gallagher EJ. Current management of migraine in US emergency departments: an analysis of the National Hospital Ambulatory Medical Care Survey. Cephalalgia. 2015;35:301–9.
11. Lipton RB, Bigal ME, Diamond M, Freitag F, Reed ML, Stewart WF; for the American Migraine Prevalence and Prevention Advisory Group. Migraine prevalence, disease burden, and the need for preventive therapy. Neurology. 2007;68:343–9.
12. Silberstein SD, Holland S, Freitag F, Dodick DW, Argoff C, Ashman C. Evidence-based guideline update: pharmacologic treatment for episodic migraine prevention in adults: report of the Quality Standards Subcommittee of the American Academy of Neurology and the American Headache Society. Neurology. 2012;78:1337–45.
13. Holland S, Silberstein SD, Freitag F, Dodick DW, Argoff C, Ashman C. Evidence-based guideline update: NSAIDs and other complementary treatments for episodic migraine prevention in adults: report of the Quality Standards Subcommittee of the American Academy of Neurology and the American Headache Society. Neurology. 2012;78:1337–45.
14. Jackson JL, Kuriyama A, Hayashino Y. Botulinum toxin A for prophylactic treatment of migraine and tension headaches in adults. JAMA. 2012;307:1736–45.
15. Blumenfeld A, Silberstein SD, Dodick DW, Aurora SK, Turkel CC, Binder WJ. Method of injection of onabotulinumtoxinA for chronic migraine: a safe, well-tolerated, and effective treatment paradigm based on the PREEMPT clinical program. Headache. 2010;50:1406–18.
16. Karsan N, Goadsby PJ. CGRP mechanism antagonists and migraine management. Curr Neurol Neurosci Rep. 2015;15:25.
17. Ho TW, Conner KM, Zhang Y, et al. Randomized controlled trial of the CGRP receptor antagonist telcagepant for migraine prevention. Neurology. 2014;83:958–66.
18. Dodick DW, Goadsby PJ, Silberstein SD, Lipton RB, Olesen J, Ashina M, et al. Safety and efficacy of ALD403, an antibody to

calcitonin gene-related peptide, for the prevention of frequent episodic migraine: a randomised, double-blind, placebo-controlled, exploratory phase 2 trial. Lancet Neurol. 2014;13:1100–7.
19. Dodick DW, Goadsby PJ, Spierings ELH, Scherer JC, Sweeney SP, Grayzel DS. Safety and efficacy of LY2951742, a monoclonal antibody to calcitonin gene-related peptide, for the prevention of migraine: a phase 2, randomised, double-blind, placebo-controlled study. Lancet Neurol. 2014;13:885–92.
20. Banzi R, Cusi C, Randazzo C, Sterzi R, Tedesco D, Moja L. Selective serotonin re-uptake inhibitors (SSRIs) and serotonin-norepinephrine reuptake inhibitors (SNRIs) for the prevention of migraine in adults (Review). Cochrane Database Syst Rev. 2015;(4):CD002919.
21. Mulleners WM, McCrory DC, Linde M. Antiepileptics in migraine prophylaxis: an updated Cochrane review. Cephalalgia. 2015;35:51–62.
22. Lipton RB, Dodick DW, Silberstein SD, Saper JR, Aurora SK, Pearlman SH, et al. Single-pulse transcranial magnetic stimulation for acute treatment of migraine with aura: a randomised, double-blind, parallel-group, sham-controlled trial. Lancet Neurol. 2010;9:373–80.
23. Dodick DW, Schembri CT, Helmuth M, Aurora SK. Transcranial magnetic stimulation for migraine: a safety review. Headache. 2010;50:1153–63.
24. Ashkenazi A, Blumenfeld A, Napchan U, Narouze S, Grosberg B, Nett R, et al. Peripheral nerve blocks and trigger point injections in headache management: a systematic review and suggestions for future research. Headache. 2010;50:943–52.
25. Chen YF, Bramley G, Unwin G, Hanu-Cernat D, Dretzke J, Moore D, et al. Occipital nerve stimulation for chronic migraine: a systematic review and meta-analysis. PLoS One. 2015;10:e0116786.
26. Diener HC, Bingel U. Surgical treatments for migraine: time to fight against the knife. Cephalalgia. 2015;35:465–8.
27. Dowson A, Mullen MJ, Peatfield R, Muir K, Khan AA, Wells C, et al. Migraine Intervention With STARFlex Technology (MIST) trial: a prospective, multicenter, double-blind, sham-controlled trial to evaluate the effectiveness of patent foramen ovale closure with STARFlex septal repair implant to resolve refractory migraine headache. Circulation. 2008;117:1397–404.

Chapter 5
Nonpharmacologic Treatment of Migraine

5.1 Introduction

Migraine and headache-related disability are exacerbated by lifestyle and behavioral factors and, accordingly, some nonpharmacologic interventions also have strong efficacy as preventive treatments. Nonpharmacologic treatments are typically used in conjunction with, rather than instead of, migraine pharmacotherapy, and large comparative trials demonstrate that adding behavioral therapies to pharmacotherapy produces outcomes superior to either intervention alone.

As discussed earlier, all patients with headache should be given basic counseling on the importance of obtaining sufficient and consistent sleep, healthy and regular eating, and limiting stress. Many patients will also benefit from a more involved nonpharmacologic intervention that provides a programmatic approach to altering physiology and behaviors that perpetuate migraine. Nonpharmacologic interventions are indicated for those with:

- Preference for nondrug treatment
- Contraindication for drug treatment (medical, pregnancy, nursing)

T.A. Smitherman, *Clinician's Manual on Migraine*,
DOI 10.1007/978-3-319-02777-7_5,

- Inadequate response to (or poor tolerance for) pharmacotherapy
- Poor adherence to current or past treatment regimens
- History of overusing acute medications or active medication overuse headache (MOH)
- Considerable life stress or poor coping skills
- Significant psychiatric comorbidity
- Past positive response to nondrug intervention for another condition
- Internal locus of control and/or high self-efficacy for managing headache

Patients with a poor or incomplete response to preventive pharmacotherapy are also excellent candidates, in which case they typically maintain a preventive medication regimen while simultaneously undergoing behavioral treatment. Interventions emphasizing development of active coping skills are often particularly well suited for patients with an internal locus of control (LOC), because they already acknowledge that they can exert some control over their headache attacks and how they respond to them.

5.2 Behavioral Therapies with Strong Empirical Support

The most well-established nonpharmacologic treatments for migraine undoubtedly are the behavioral therapies of progressive muscle relaxation, biofeedback, and stress management training. When administered in combination, which is the typical mode of delivery in clinical settings, these interventions are often referred to as cognitive behavioral therapy (CBT). Collectively, these treatments are generally equivalent to the common preventive medications in reducing migraine frequency, as established in dozens of studies and numerous meta-analyses of controlled trials over the past 40 years [1]. These interventions typically yield reductions in headache frequency of 35–55 %, similar to outcomes obtained from the efficacious preventive pharmacotherapies. Long-term follow-up studies indicate that most patients maintain their treatment gains for years after therapy ends. Moreover, these interventions are cost-effective, even when compared to the most inexpensive preventive pharmacotherapies [2].

The strong evidence for these behavioral therapies culminated in them being designated as having Grade A evidence for migraine prevention by the United States Headache Consortium [3]. Multiple large-scale randomized controlled trials have since demonstrated that adding behavioral treatment to preventive pharmacotherapy results in better outcomes than either treatment alone, both for adults and children/adolescents with migraine [4, 5]. This level of evidence for the increased efficacy resulting from combining behavioral and pharmacologic therapies would now also be considered Grade A.

The behavioral migraine therapies described below typically are administered by psychologists and other professionals with graduate training in principles of behavior change. Treatment sessions typically occur weekly for 2–3 months, although "limited-contact" treatments requiring only a few in-office sessions have similar efficacy as long as patients are willing to learn and practice the skills independently. Biofeedback requires more technical skill and familiarity with psychophysiology than other behavioral therapies and thus should be carried out by an individual who has received supervised training in biofeedback.

5.2.1 Progressive Muscle Relaxation

Progressive muscle relaxation (PMR) is a programmatic method for teaching muscular relaxation that first involves tensing then releasing various muscle groups in a sequential fashion. The rationale for PMR is that relaxation reduces sympathetic nervous system arousal that often precedes headache and that patients can become proficient in both noticing and reducing this arousal with regular practice.

Patients are taught the basic procedures and sequences of tensing/releasing muscles and instructed in the importance of daily practice for skill development and generalization. As proficiency with the initial 16-muscle group series develops, these 16 groups are consolidated into 7 muscle groups, then 4 muscle groups, and then into "relaxation by recall" without the need for sequential tensing. The importance of daily practice cannot be overemphasized, and many patients will not notice significant improvement during the initial few weeks of practicing PMR. (As with preventive medications, patients should be advised on regular adherence regardless of initial results, because they may otherwise stop treatment if benefits are not immediately apparent.)

5.2.2 Biofeedback

Biofeedback has a long history in the field of behavioral medicine. Biofeedback involves teaching the patient to deliberately alter autonomic physiological processes normally considered outside of voluntary control. With migraine, biofeedback is typically thermal (increasing body temperature) or electromyographic (reducing scalp muscle tension) in nature. Both forms of biofeedback are efficacious for migraine prevention, and blood volume pulse biofeedback also has demonstrated efficacy but is used less commonly. In clinic settings, biofeedback systems commonly involve computerized equipment that feed back to the patient auditory and/or visual stimuli indicative of success. With continued practice, patients learn gradual control over sympathetic arousal. Children may benefit even more from biofeedback than adult headache patients do, as many enjoy biofeedback training that involves displays resembling video or computer games.

5.2.3 Stress and Trigger Management Training

Stress management involves teaching patients to recognize stressors and implement problem-focused coping skills to manage them. The stressors of interest are those that occur frequently and that often precede headache onset (e.g., argument with a loved one, a work deadline, family gatherings). Patients are taught to avoid stressors for which avoidance is feasible, to better manage those that cannot always be avoided (e.g., family stress, work deadlines) through active coping skills, and to prepare for those that can be predicted but not prevented (e.g., weather events, menstruation). Stress management is usually administered in conjunction with PMR or biofeedback.

Because the skills of self-monitoring and managing stress apply similarly to other precipitants of headache (e.g., missing meals, changes in sleep, diet, menstruation), often patients are counseled in basic strategies of identifying and managing other headache triggers.

5.2.4 Other Behavioral Interventions

In addition to these well-established behavioral treatments, other behavioral interventions such as acceptance and commitment therapy (ACT) and mindfulness appear promising, but their body of efficacy is more limited as a function of small clinical trials [6]. Components of these interventions may prove valuable for patients who respond insufficiently to standard migraine treatments, but at present they cannot be recommended as first-line interventions until further studies are conducted.

In addition to the promise of ACT and mindfulness for migraine, studies are emerging suggesting that behavioral treatment for common migraine comorbidities may improve migraine. The data are strongest at present for insomnia, with two small randomized, placebo-controlled trials showing that behavioral treatment of insomnia holds promise for reducing migraine frequency among individuals with CM [7, 8]. Similarly, research efforts to study the efficacy of behavioral weight loss programs in reducing migraine are underway.

5.3 Referrals for Behavioral Therapy

Despite their strong efficacy for migraine, primary care providers infrequently refer migraine patients for behavioral headache therapies [9], in part because many are unaware of the evidence base or unsure how to make such a referral.

The referring provider should endeavor to refer patients to mental health clinicians who have expertise working with medical patients, the associated disciplines of which are commonly referred to as "health psychology" and "behavioral medicine." Most mental health providers with a background in behavioral medicine are proficient with the interventions of PMR, CBT, and behavior modification, even if they do not regularly treat patients with headache. Table 5.1 provides resources for locating behavioral providers and treatment information.

In addition to identifying a qualified behavioral provider, the referring clinician should briefly educate the patient about the reason for making the referral, as too frequently patients present for behavioral treatment without understanding why they were referred in the first place. The main points of emphasis should be that behavioral therapies are intended to supplement (not replace) pharmacotherapy, the best outcomes are achieved when patients receive both pharmacotherapy and behavioral treatment, and a patient is not referred to a behavioral therapist because a clinician believes they are mentally ill or fabricating their symptoms. Clinicians should seek to normalize emotional reactions to chronic pain (e.g., stress, mood changes, anxiety) and help the patient make the connection between how her own behaviors influence migraine (e.g., high stress, poor sleep, eating habits). Additionally, clinicians should emphasize that the focus of behavioral headache treatments is not principally to address mental health but instead to help patients learn ways to modify specific behaviors in order to reduce their migraine attacks and improve coping skills. Patients should be reminded that behavioral interventions for

TABLE 5.1 Resources for locating behavioral providers and treatment information

Well-established behavioral therapies for migraine prevention	Relaxation training Thermal biofeedback plus relaxation training Electromyographic biofeedback Cognitive–behavioral therapy Stress management
Visiting a behavioral therapist	Association for Behavioral and Cognitive Therapies "Find a Therapist" function (www.abct.org) Biofeedback Certification International Alliance "Find a Practitioner" function (www.bcia.org) Association for Applied Psychophysiology and Biofeedback "Find a Practitioner" function (www.aapb.org)
Information for clinicians about behavioral migraine treatments	Treatment guide and patient handouts [10] Reimbursement and billing codes (for US-based providers) [11].
Information for clinicians and patients about behavioral migraine treatments	American Migraine Foundation European Headache Foundation The Migraine Trust International Headache Society

migraine are designed to be short term in nature, require office visits for 2–3 months, and are part of a multidisciplinary treatment plan.

5.4 Other Nonpharmacologic Interventions

Several nonpharmacologic treatments with widespread name recognition are not well established for treating migraine, including yoga, acupuncture, and chiropractic manipulation.

Though some small trials or clinical anecdotes have reported positive results, very few controlled studies have been conducted on these interventions as preventive treatments for migraine. Most existing studies suffer from small sample sizes, equivalence to sham controls, and mixed findings, and thus, these interventions should not be considered as first- or second-line treatment options at present.

References

1. Rains JC, Penzien DB, McCrory DC, Gray RN. Behavioral headache treatment: history, review of the empirical literature, and methodological critique. Headache. 2005;45 suppl 2:S92–109.
2. Schafer AM, Rains JC, Penzien DB, Groban L, Smitherman TA, Houle TT. Direct costs of preventive headache treatments: comparison of behavioral and pharmacologic agents. Headache. 2011;51:985–91.
3. Silberstein SD, for the US Headache Consortium. Practice parameter: evidence-based guidelines for migraine headache (an evidence-based review): report of the Quality Standards Subcommittee of the American Academy of Neurology. Neurology. 2000;55:754–63.
4. Holroyd KA, Cottrell CK, O'Donnell FJ, Cordingley GE, Drew JB, Carlson BW, et al. Effect of preventive (beta blocker) treatment, behavioural migraine management, or their combination on outcomes of optimised acute treatment in frequent migraine: randomised controlled trial. BMJ. 2010;341:c4871.
5. Powers SW, Kashikar-Zuck SM, Allen JR, LeCates SL, Slater SK, Zafar M, et al. Cognitive behavioral therapy plus amitriptyline for chronic migraine in children and adolescents: a randomized clinical trial. JAMA. 2013;310:2622–30.
6. Smitherman TA, Wells RE, Ford SG. Emerging behavioral treatments for migraine. Curr Pain Headache Rep. 2015;19:486.
7. Calhoun AH, Ford S. Behavioral sleep modification may revert transformed migraine to episodic migraine. Headache. 2007;47:1178–83.
8. Smitherman TA. Walters AB, Davis RE, et al. Randomized controlled trial of behavioral insomnia treatment for chronic migraine with comorbid insomnia. Headache. 2016;56:276–91.

9. Minen MT, Loder E, Tishler L, Silbersweig D. Migraine diagnosis and treatment: a knowledge and needs assessment among primary care providers. Cephalalgia. 2016;36:358–70.
10. Smitherman TA, Penzien DB, Rains JC, Nicholson R, Houle TT. Headache. Cambridge, MA: Hogrefe; 2015.
11. American Psychological Association (APA). Health and behavior codes. www.apapracticecentral.org/reimbursement/billing/. Accessed 29 March 2016.

MIX
Papier aus verantwortungsvollen Quellen
Paper from responsible sources
FSC® C105338

If you have any concerns about our products,
you can contact us on
ProductSafety@springernature.com

In case Publisher is established outside the EU,
the EU authorized representative is:
Springer Nature Customer Service Center GmbH
Europaplatz 3, 69115 Heidelberg, Germany

Printed by Libri Plureos GmbH
in Hamburg, Germany